EMERGENCY INFORMATION

Emergency Medical Phone Number - 911
or
Local Emergency Medical Number - _____

INFORMATION NEEDED

Address: _____

Cross Streets: _____

Phone Number: _____

Emergency Situation: _____

Number of Persons Needing Help: _____

Condition of Victim(s): _____

What is being done (e.g., CPR): _____

DO NOT HANG UP UNTIL THE PERSON
YOU CALLED HANGS UP FIRST!

YOU ARE IT:
FIRST AID

When Minutes Count

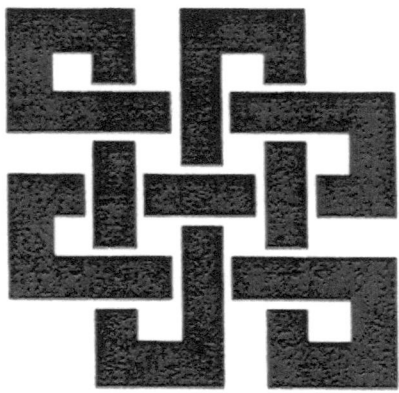

BEVERLY J. COFFMAN, R.N., B.S.N.
GUNNAR G. SEVELIUS, M.D.

With Foreword By:
DONALD TRUNKEY, M.D.

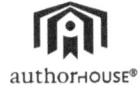

authorHOUSE®

AuthorHouse™
1663 Liberty Drive, Suite 200
Bloomington, IN 47403
www.authorhouse.com
Phone: 1-800-839-8640

First published by AuthorHouse 1/20/2009

ISBN: 978-1-4343-9797-3 (sc)

Printed in the United States of America
Bloomington, Indiana

This book is printed on acid-free paper.

OTHER BOOKS BY THE AUTHOR:

Add Years to Your Life and Life to Your Years:

  Volume I: Heart Attack Prevention

  Volume II: Family and Work Enhancement

The Nine Pillars of History: An Anthropological Review of History, Five Religions and Sexuality

Radioisotopes and Circulation

IN SWEDISH:

Historiens Nio Grundstenar: Även en Guide för Världsfred

*The eternal loop pictured on the cover
is an old Asian sign for longevity.*

YOU ARE IT: FIRST AID

When Minutes Count

BEVERLY J. COFFMAN, R.N., B.S.N.
GUNNAR G. SEVELIUS, M.D.

with Foreword by:
DONALD TRUNKEY, M.D.

You must give some time to your fellow man. Even if it's a little thing, do something for those who have need of help, something for which you get no pay but the privilege of doing it.

— Dr. Albert Schweitzer

TABLE OF CONTENTS

Unit   **Page**

FOREWORD

This booklet is timely and important. It could save your life or prevent permanent disability. Each day thousands of Americans suffer life-threatening illness or injury and many will die. In many instances, their deaths could be prevented if simple first aid had been initiated prior to the arrival of medical help. This booklet outlines the simple things *you* can do until medical help arrives or the victim can be taken to the nearest *appropriate* health facility.

Although the booklet is not a substitute for a comprehensive first aid or CPR course, it does present a succinct review that represents the consensus of many physicians. If you have doubts about any of the content, consult your own doctor. Remember, you are responsible for your own health and you can help others if you know the contents of this booklet.

— Donald D. Trunkey, M.D
Chief of Surgery, San Francisco General Hospital

This booklet presents procedures that can help victims in medical emergencies. Although the procedures outlined are commonly used, other possibilities do exist and should be discussed with one's physician. Because most of these emergencies are life threatening, the first person at the scene can often be of tremendous assistance before profes-sional help arrives. It is strongly recommended, however, that any person giving assistance evaluate the situation to ascertain whether he or she may be of assistance, keeping in mind that some kinds of problems may not be covered in the booklet and that there is no guarantee that one's actions will be successful.

— Gunnar Sevelius, M.D.

INTRODUCTION

Every day thousands of people are faced with emergency medical situations that demand immediate action to prevent death or permanent injury. Even in a large industrial plant having its own ambulance service, the professional medical people rarely can reach the emergency scene in less than five minutes. Experience has shown, however, that, in cases requiring cardiopulmonary resuscitation, great success has occurred when about every tenth employee has been trained in CPR. These employees are so close to their coworkers that they can help immediately in time of medical emergency. Even if professionals are close by, experience has shown that there is a need for the average person to know how to handle certain medical emergencies until professional help arrives.

This booklet was written with that in mind. Statistics from a local emergency department were used to determine which situations to include in the book. Seventeen medical emergencies in which untrained people could deliver help of utmost importance were selected for this booklet. The sequence of the units reflects the importance of immediate action. The flow charts will help you determine the order of the action to be taken, and we have included the Emergency Medical Services (EMS) number (911) when appropriate, to aid you in getting professional help. The emergency information at the front of the book should be posted near your phone so that you can send for help quickly. Take the time to write down the necessary information. Include the TTY emergency phone number (found in the front of your phone book) on the list if there are people with a hearing impairment in your family.

A very important component of the booklet is the *prevention tips*. You may also add your own tips to personalize them for you. "An ounce of prevention is worth many pounds of cure."

This booklet is valuable as a quick reference, and is not meant to take the place of formal training in first aid and CPR. These classes are available through industry, American Red Cross, American Heart Association, local colleges and hospitals.

A well-stocked first aid kit increases your ability to act fast when faced with an emergency situation. If the one you purchase does not have the following items, it would be wise to add them: (a) sterile eye dropper, (b) small bulb syringe, (c) one-ounce bottle of ipecac for every child in home (keep out of children's reach), (d) eye patch, (e) six-ounce paper cup, and (f) snakebite kit.

Last, but not least, we hope you never have to use the information in this booklet. However, if you do have the opportunity to help someone and you do it well, we promise you a soaring joy that can only be felt by those who have saved a person's life or prevented someone from having a permanent injury.

Acknowledgements: Special thanks to Dr. Donald Trunkey, Chief of Surgery, San Francisco General Hospital, and Professor of Surgery, University of California, San Francisco, for his review and endorsement of our effort. Dr. Trunkey is recognized as a national authority on trauma medicine and emergency medical treatment, and has been an important advocate of shortening the time between a medical emergency and definitive medical treatment. Many thanks also to Dr. Sevelius' secretary, Gloria Braman, and to Technical Publications, Lockheed Astronautics Division.

HOW TO USE FLOW CHARTS

The flow charts in this booklet will aid you in discerning appropriate actions quickly. Become familiar with the symbols and flow charts so that your evaluation can be accurate and your actions effective.

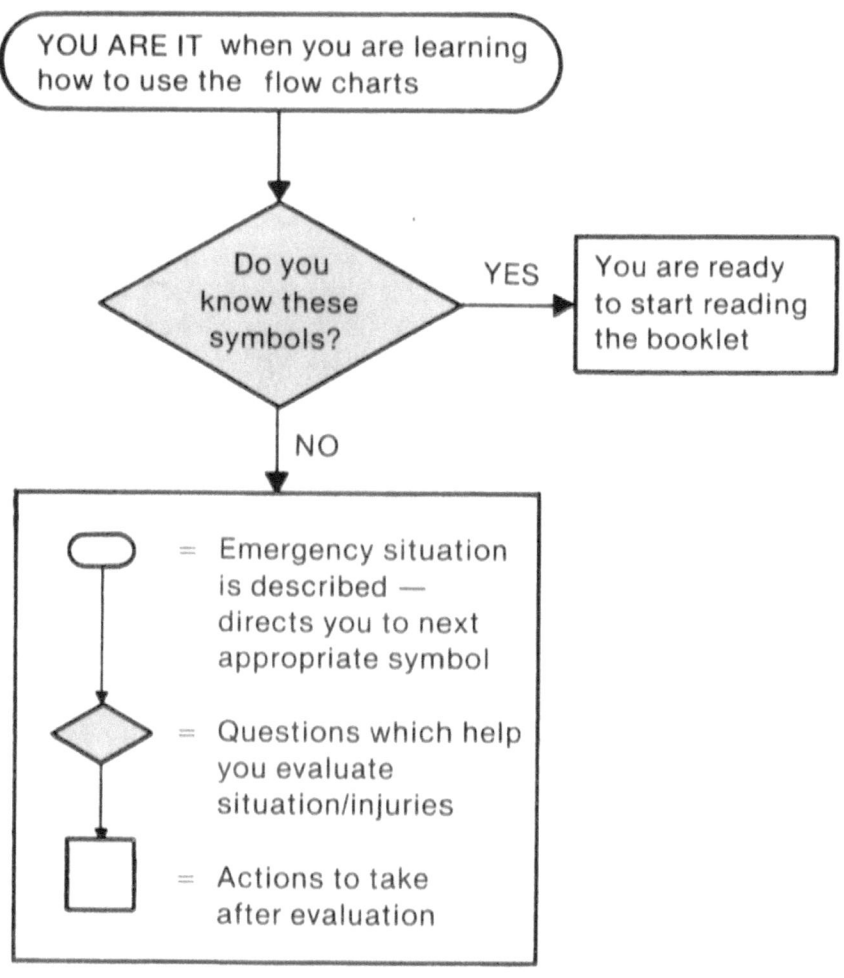

SETTING PRIORITIES FOR EMERGENCY CARE WHEN YOU ARE IT

Whenever an accident occurs there is a possibility of life-threatening problems. Therefore it is important to know how to check the accident victim and quickly prioritize your actions when giving first aid.

In all emergency situations, the most important considerations are to ensure (a) a safe environment (i.e., removing victim from a fire, or room full of carbon monoxide or smoke), (b) an open airway, (c) adequate breathing, (d) adequate circulation, and (e) an appropriate call for help.

The ABCs of cardiopulmonary resuscitation (CPR) is an effective tool to remind you of the initial assessment actions. An automatic recall of these steps can be maintained by using a visualization technique when doing routine activities which require no thought, i.e., doing dishes, exercising, etc. *Visualize* a person falling from a ladder and then all the actions needed to care for him. Vary the circumstances so that you experience different actions which might be needed.

PREVENTION TIPS:

It is extremely important for *everyone* to be proficient in administering CPR. The technical skills and knowledge required for administering CPR are easy to learn and maintain when a valid course in CPR is taken. Courses which lead to certification in CPR are offered by the American Heart Association, American Red Cross, some community colleges, some hospitals and some workplaces.

Don't be a helpless bystander; prepare yourself before tragedy strikes. Your actions could save someone you love.

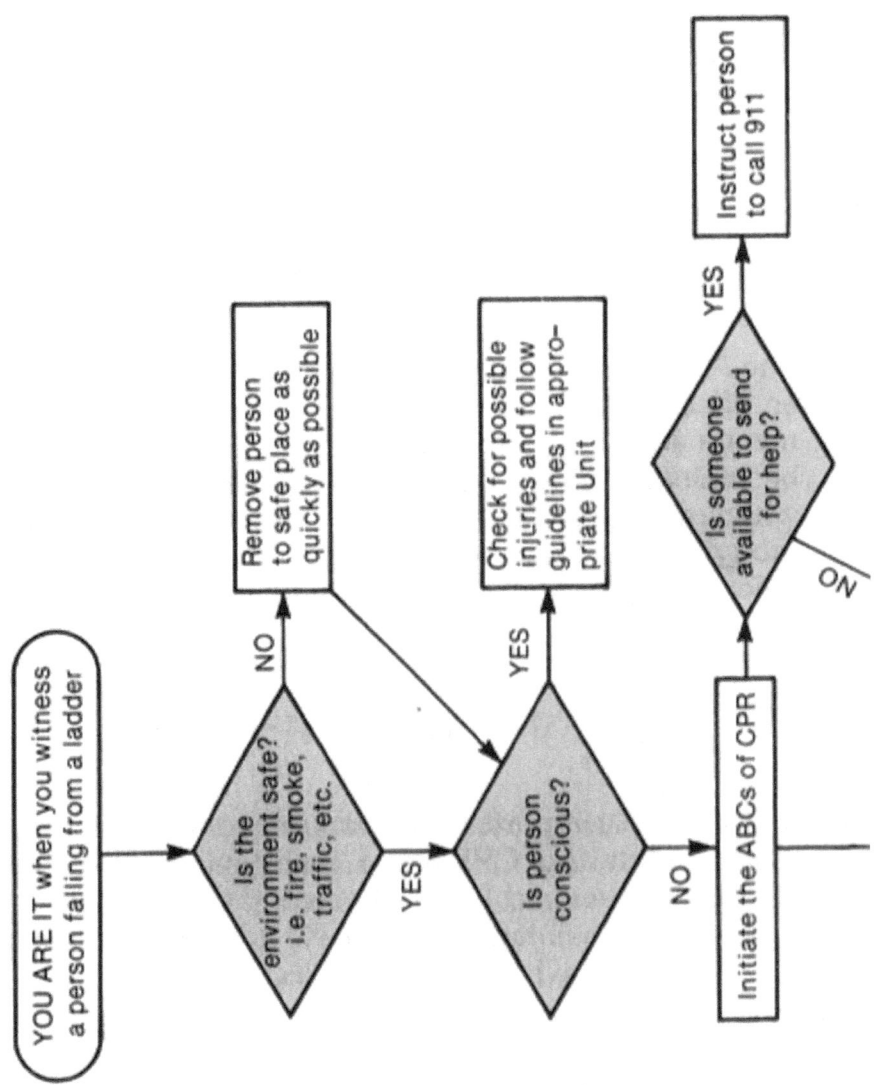

YOU ARE IT when you witness a person falling from a ladder

Is the environment safe? i.e. fire, smoke, traffic, etc.

NO → Remove person to safe place as quickly as possible

YES

Is person conscious?

YES → Check for possible injuries and follow guidelines in appro—priate Unit

NO

Initiate the ABCs of CPR

Is someone available to send for help?

YES → Instruct person to call 911

NO

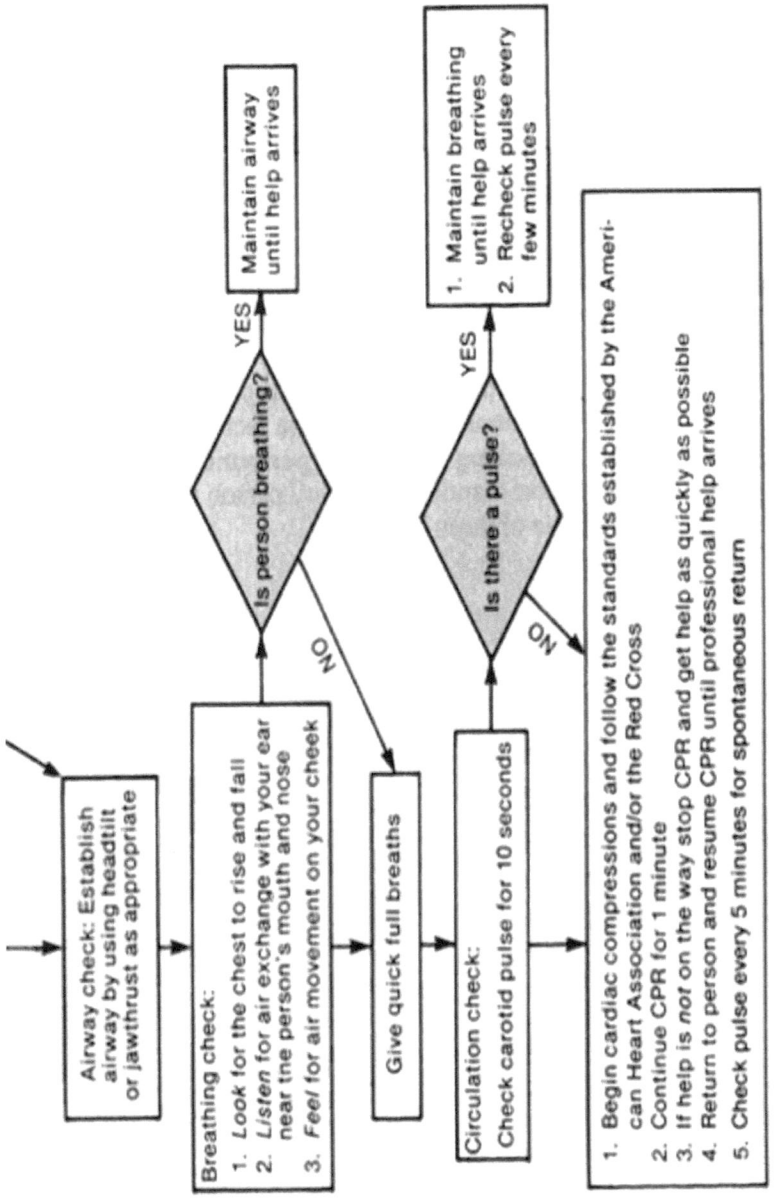

Airway check: Establish airway by using headtilt or jawthrust as appropriate

Breathing check:
1. *Look* for the chest to rise and fall
2. *Listen* for air exchange with your ear near the person's mouth and nose
3. *Feel* for air movement on your cheek

Is person breathing?

YES — Maintain airway until help arrives

NO

Give quick full breaths

Circulation check:
Check carotid pulse for 10 seconds

Is there a pulse?

YES
1. Maintain breathing until help arrives
2. Recheck pulse every few minutes

NO

1. Begin cardiac compressions and follow the standards established by the American Heart Association and/or the Red Cross
2. Continue CPR for 1 minute
3. If help is *not* on the way stop CPR and get help as quickly as possible
4. Return to person and resume CPR until professional help arrives
5. Check pulse every 5 minutes for spontaneous return

EMERGENCY CARE FOR CHOKING WHEN YOU ARE IT

Each year thousands of Americans die from choking, even though a method to treat the choking victim is easy and effective, when learned correctly. Classes are available through the American Heart Association, American Red Cross, some Community Colleges, some hospitals, and some workplaces. Since severe complications can occur if the techniques for treating the choking victim are performed incorrectly, it is recommended that every person take advantage of one of these classes.

PREVENTION TIPS:

- Make sure food, especially meat, is cut into small pieces
- Chew food slowly and thoroughly
- Do not laugh and/or talk excessively when eating
- Do not drink alcohol excessively before or during meals
- Do not allow children to walk, run or play with objects or food in their mouths
- Keep small objects (i.e., buttons, marbles, etc.) away from infants and small children
- Be sure infant has ability to handle solid food before offering it
- Become certified in CPR

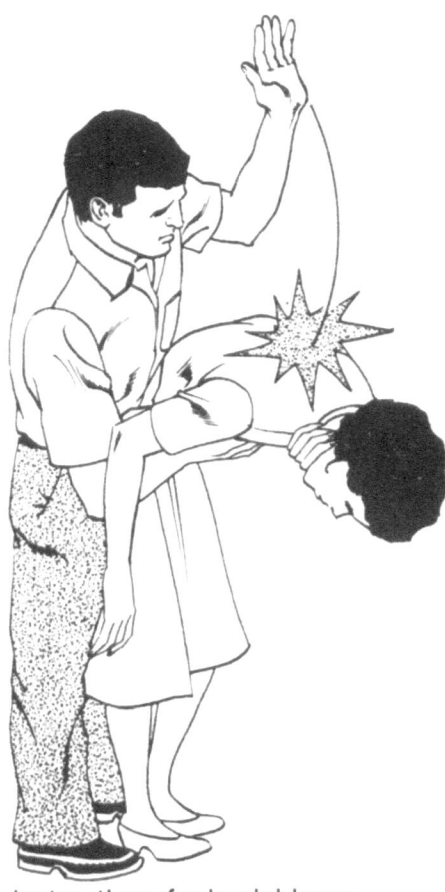

For Instructions, refer to flow chart on next page.

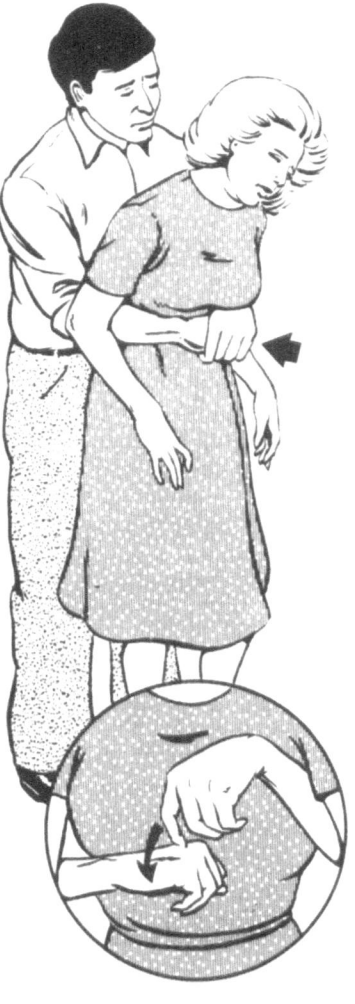

Instructions for back blows:
- Stand behind the victim, and place one hand on her chest for support
- Lean her forward so that her head is at chest level or lower
- Quickly deliver four sharp blows between shoulder blades with the heel of your hand

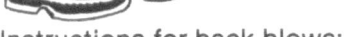

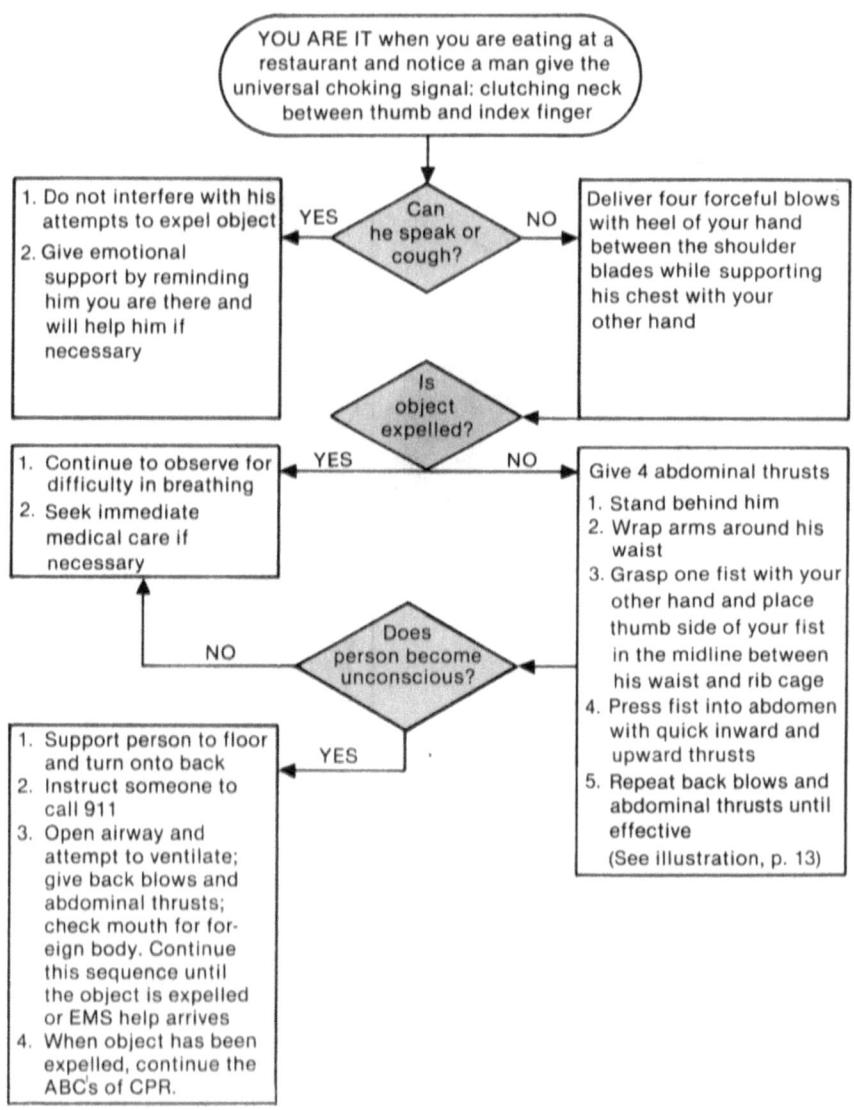

YOU ARE IT when you are eating at a restaurant and notice a man give the universal choking signal: clutching neck between thumb and index finger

Can he speak or cough?

YES →
1. Do not interfere with his attempts to expel object
2. Give emotional support by reminding him you are there and will help him if necessary

NO → Deliver four forceful blows with heel of your hand between the shoulder blades while supporting his chest with your other hand

Is object expelled?

YES →
1. Continue to observe for difficulty in breathing
2. Seek immediate medical care if necessary

NO → Give 4 abdominal thrusts
1. Stand behind him
2. Wrap arms around his waist
3. Grasp one fist with your other hand and place thumb side of your fist in the midline between his waist and rib cage
4. Press fist into abdomen with quick inward and upward thrusts
5. Repeat back blows and abdominal thrusts until effective
(See illustration, p. 13)

Does person become unconscious?

NO (→ back to "Continue to observe")

YES →
1. Support person to floor and turn onto back
2. Instruct someone to call 911
3. Open airway and attempt to ventilate; give back blows and abdominal thrusts; check mouth for foreign body. Continue this sequence until the object is expelled or EMS help arrives
4. When object has been expelled, continue the ABC's of CPR.

EMERGENCY CARE FOR NEAR DROWNING WHEN YOU ARE IT

Death due to drowning is especially sad because irresponsible behavior is usually involved in the tragedy. It is best to prevent drowning by following the prevention tips. However, when near drowning does occur, effective use of CPR skills is essential. Have you learned, and are you maintaining CPR skills? (See Unit 1 for finding available classes.) Each year thousands of people die due to drowning. Will you be able to help them if *you are it?*

Frequently, a near drowning victim will start to breathe at the scene of the accident. Even so, the victim should be taken to the nearest emergency room without delay. Complications, resulting from a change in body chemistry due to swallowing or inhaling a large amount of salt or fresh water, might not be apparent for the first 24 to 72 hours. The medical team will run tests which will detect complications in the early stages before devastating effects have a chance to develop.

PREVENTION TIPS:

- Know CPR
- Never allow young children near *any* water (even bathtubs) without *adult* supervision
- Know your swimming ability, never try to go beyond it, and never swim alone
- When swimming in unfamiliar waters, be aware of and avoid areas of plant growth which might entangle or trap you
- Never dive into water before investigating its depth and the presence of hazardous objects such as rocks
- When swimming in rivers or the ocean, be aware of currents, undercurrents and riptides

- Do not drink alcoholic beverages while participating in water sports such as boating, skiing, swimming, etc. (One-third of all adult deaths due to drowning involve the consumption of alcoholic beverages)

- Never take in a series of deep, fast breaths before swimming underwater. (The decrease in your body's CO_2 will tell your brain that you do not need to breathe until you are unconscious and unable to surface)

- Never try to rescue another person if it will endanger your own life; use extreme caution when approaching a drowning victim in the water. (The person may panic and pull both of you down)

- Use U.S. Coast Guard approved life jackets when boating, even though you are a strong swimmer. (If there is a boating accident, you might become unconscious)

- Know and follow safety rules when boating

- Use a pole or throw rope to person

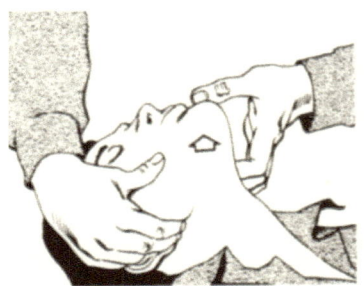

If neck injury is suspected, do not tilt the head. Open the airway by placing the tips of your index and middle fingers on the corners of the victim's jaw to lift it forward, thus moving the tongue away from the back of the throat.

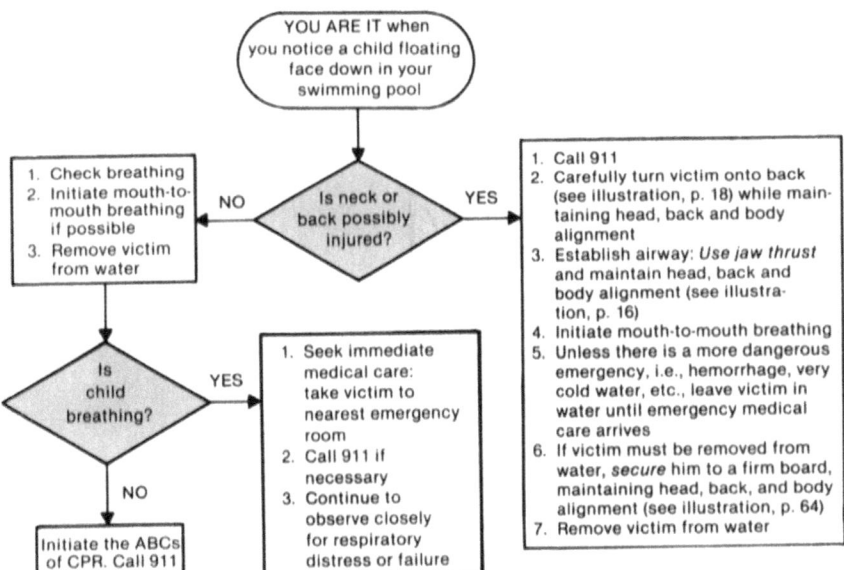

YOU ARE IT when you notice a child floating face down in your swimming pool

Is neck or back possibly injured?

NO
1. Check breathing
2. Initiate mouth-to-mouth breathing if possible
3. Remove victim from water

YES
1. Call 911
2. Carefully turn victim onto back (see illustration, p. 18) while maintaining head, back and body alignment
3. Establish airway: *Use jaw thrust* and maintain head, back and body alignment (see illustration, p. 16)
4. Initiate mouth-to-mouth breathing
5. Unless there is a more dangerous emergency, i.e., hemorrhage, very cold water, etc., leave victim in water until emergency medical care arrives
6. If victim must be removed from water, *secure* him to a firm board, maintaining head, back, and body alignment (see illustration, p. 64)
7. Remove victim from water

Is child breathing?

YES
1. Seek immediate medical care: take victim to nearest emergency room
2. Call 911 if necessary
3. Continue to observe closely for respiratory distress or failure

NO
Initiate the ABCs of CPR. Call 911

Important CPR Reminders
- Do not attempt to remove water from the stomach, unless it interferes with respiration
- Evaluate person for neck and/or back injury, and use jaw thrust rather than head tilt if appropriate
- Mouth-to-mouth breathing should be started in the water if it does not endanger the life of the victim or the rescuer
- Do not attempt to remove water from the lungs (Water inhaled into the lungs is absorbed by the body very quickly)

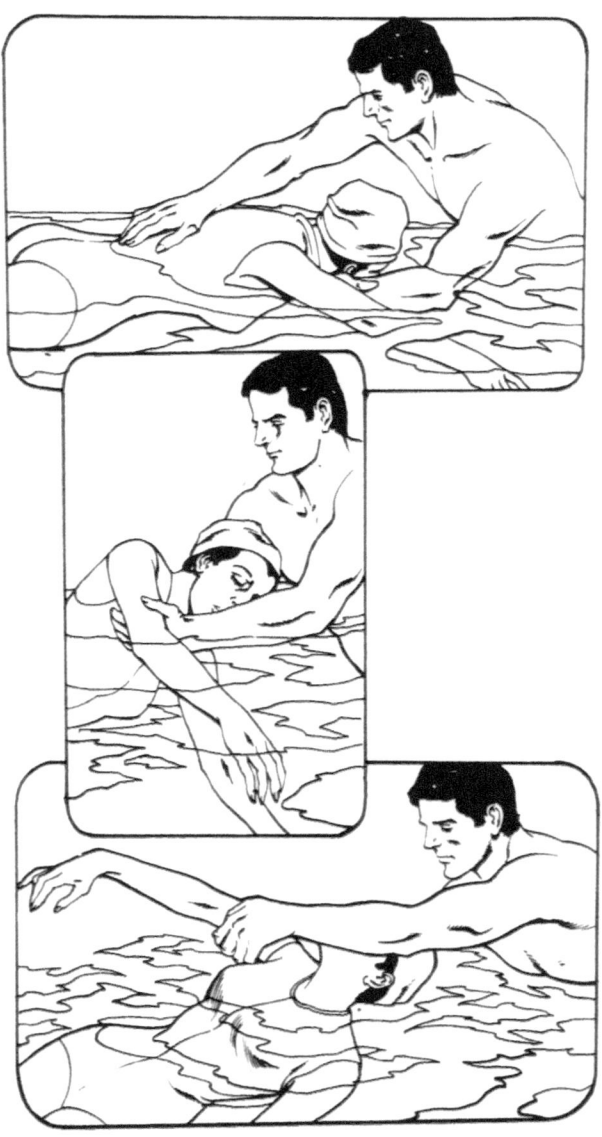

Turn the victim over while maintaining alignment of head and body. Place one hand in the middle of victim's back keeping your arm over her head. Put your other hand under the victim's upper arm close to her shoulder. Maintaining head and body alignment, rotate her by lifting her shoulder up and over.

EMERGENCY CARE FOR CHEST PAIN/ HEART ATTACK WHEN YOU ARE IT

Every year thousands of Americans, in every walk of life, die from a heart attack. Fifty percent of all heart attack victims die before reaching the hospital emergency room. Many of these people could have been saved if immediate, efficient, effective home emergency care had been available to them.

Heart attacks occur when the blood supply to a part of the heart muscle is diminished or completely blocked. When this happens the heart does not function correctly and life is threatened. Sometimes the body's own protective mechanisms act to help the heart continue to beat. (Some of these mechanisms are responsible for the signs and symptoms of the heart attack.) However, sometimes the mechanisms fail and the heart stops. Cardiopulmonary resuscitation (CPR) is then needed until the medical team can restore the heart's action with drugs and other modern techniques.

Thus, the person suffering chest pain needs help which requires knowledge of the signs and symptoms of heart attack *and* skills in CPR. CPR techniques can be learned only by practice on a mannequin with a qualified instructor as a guide. The American Heart Association, the American Red Cross, some community colleges, some hospitals and some work places provide classes in CPR. Will you be prepared to help a person suffering chest pain?

Clinical studies have identified several health and life style factors which contribute to a higher potential for suffering a heart attack. *High blood pressure, excess body fat, lack of a routine exercise program, a smoking habit, unbalanced stress, excess serum cholesterol, and uncontrolled diabetes* are risk factors which can be controlled by the individual. Heredity, sex, age and race are factors which cannot be controlled by the individual. It is significant that the risk of heart attack increases with the aggregate number and severity of the risk factors which apply to the individual.

Also, remember that children use adults as role models. When you reduce your own risk, you also reduce a child's risk who is "looking up to you."

PREVENTION TIPS:

- Learn signs and symptoms of heart attack
- Learn and remain competent in administering CPR
- Read and follow recommendations in "Add Years to Your Life and Life to Your Years, Volume I" by Gunnar G. Sevelius

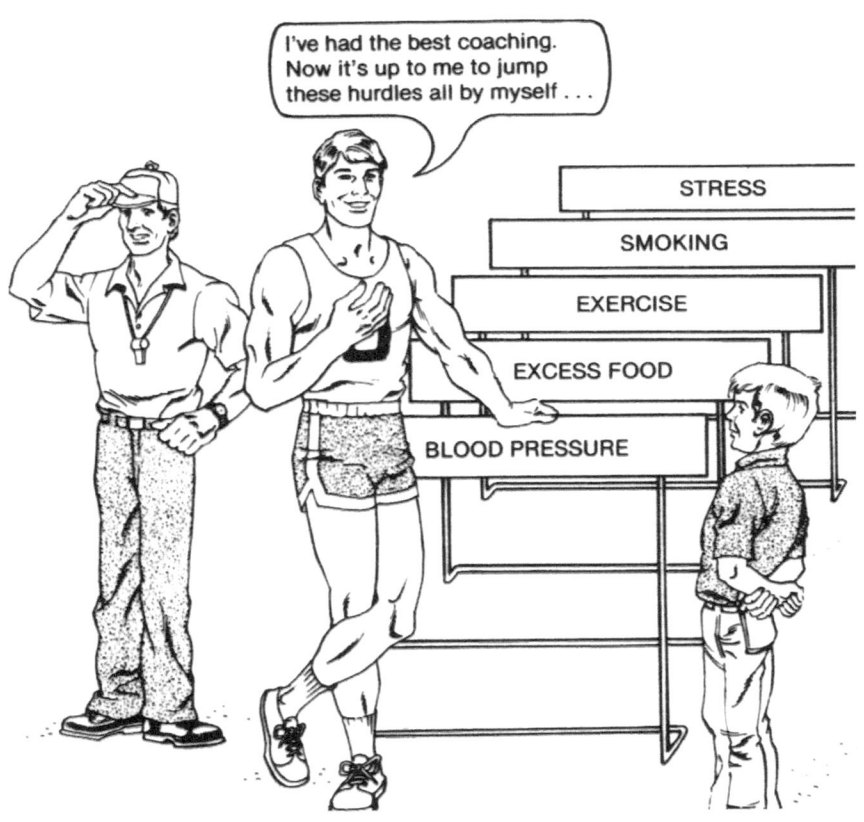

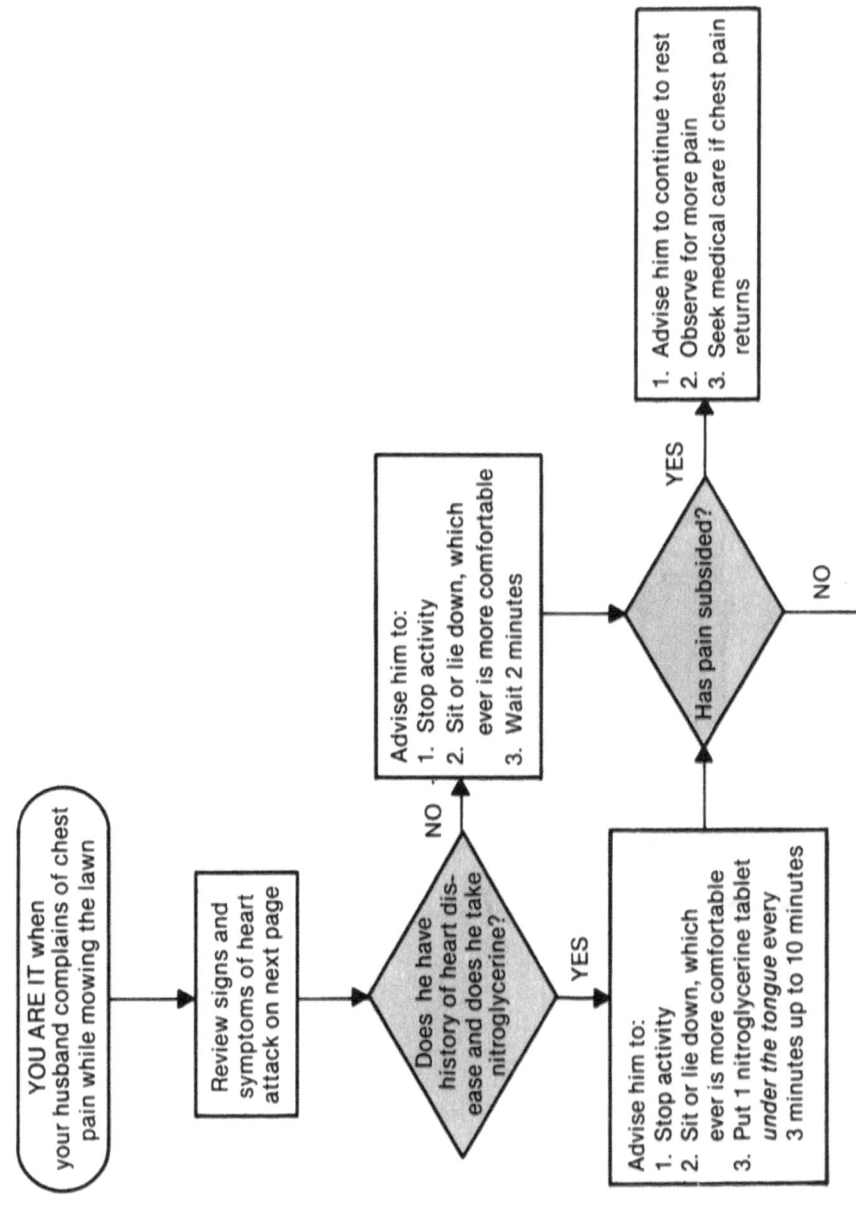

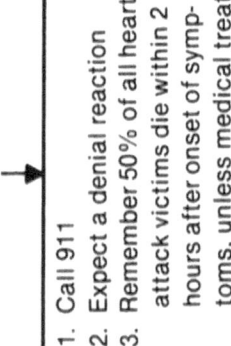

1. Call 911
2. Expect a denial reaction
3. Remember 50% of all heart attack victims die within 2 hours after onset of symptoms, unless medical treatment is given

Signs and symptoms of heart attack:

1. Chest Pain that:
   a. Is an uncomfortable pressure, squeezing or feeling of fullness in the center of the chest, behind the breast bone
   b. May spread to the shoulder(s), arm(s), neck, or jaw
   c. Lasts longer than 2 minutes after a person stops activity
   d. Is not necessarily severe
2. Sweating
3. Nausea
4. Shortness of breath
5. A feeling of weakness
6. Denial that a heart attack is a possibility

EMERGENCY CARE FOR SEVERE ALLERGIC REACTION

A severe allergic reaction (also called *anaphylaxis*) can be one of the most catastrophic, death threatening emergencies you may encounter. Rapidly obtaining emergency medical assistance is crucial if the person (1) is known to have serious allergies, and (2) is displaying severe allergic symptoms. An adrenaline injection followed by an antihistamine injection is the only available treatment for the anaphylactic reaction.

Severe allergic reactions may result in a collapse of basic life sustaining systems such as heart and lung functions. They are caused by a culprit agent to which the person has developed a hypersensitivity. Every time the person is exposed to the particular agent, a more severe reaction tends to occur. The most common agents can be divided into four groups:

- Food, e.g. shellfish, fish, strawberries and milk
- Insect venom, e.g. bees and yellow jackets
- Drugs, e.g. penicillin, aspirin, and x-ray dye (probably the most common), horse serum
- Inhaled substances, e.g. pollens, and cigarette smoke

Some people are more prone to severe allergic reactions than others. If a person has had an episode of anaphylaxis, a physician will usually prescribe an emergency allergy kit so that the person will have immediate treatment available if exposed to the allergic agent again.

PREVENTION TIPS:

If prone to severe allergies:

- Consult your physician about an emergency allergy kit, and always carry it with you

- Know what you are allergic to and avoid exposure
- Wear medic alert jewelry or cards
- When admitted to a hospital, be sure to let the health professionals know what you are allergic to

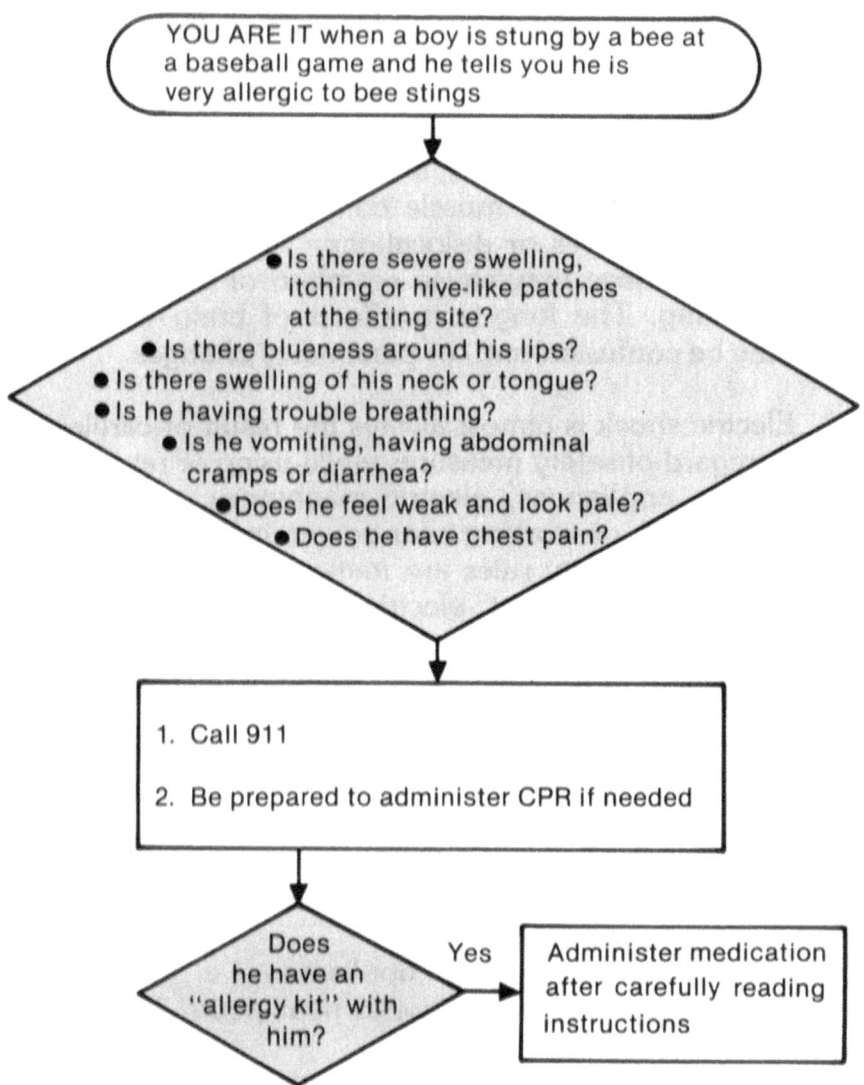

YOU ARE IT when a boy is stung by a bee at a baseball game and he tells you he is very allergic to bee stings

- Is there severe swelling, itching or hive-like patches at the sting site?
- Is there blueness around his lips?
- Is there swelling of his neck or tongue?
- Is he having trouble breathing?
- Is he vomiting, having abdominal cramps or diarrhea?
- Does he feel weak and look pale?
- Does he have chest pain?

1. Call 911

2. Be prepared to administer CPR if needed

Does he have an "allergy kit" with him?

Yes → Administer medication after carefully reading instructions

EMERGENCY CARE FOR ELECTRIC SHOCK WHEN YOU ARE IT

The effect of electric shock depends on the amount of electric current the victim is subjected to. Normal household current is strong enough to seriously injure or even kill a person. Electric shock causes violent muscle contractions, brain or nerve damage and burns. The violent muscle contractions may cause skeletal fractures or dislocations. The brain and/or nerve damage may cause cessation of the heart or breathing. The long-term effects of brain damage may be confusion and/or personality changes.

Electric shock is almost always the result of careless disregard of safety measures while using or repairing electric appliances, electric machinery, or power equipment, or working near power lines. Always insisting that safety rules are meticulously followed is the best way to "treat" electric shock.

PREVENTION TIPS:

- Disconnect electric current to *any* appliance, electric machinery or power equipment *before* attempting to repair it

- Turn off main power switch to house when working on any electrical outlets or major appliance, i.e., electric stove

- Do not use electrical appliances, i.e. hair dryers, curling irons, phones, near pools, hot tubs or saunas

- Use safety plugs in electric outlets if there are infants or small children in the home

- Do not use any electrical appliance that has a defective cord or plug

- Follow manufacturer's recommendations diligently when using electrical appliances

- Do not allow exposed electric wires to remain near any water
- Do not use electrical appliances while standing on wet or damp ground
- Use only three-prong grounded plugs for all appliances and power equipment
- When digging or working near power lines be aware of where they are and avoid touching them

Add some of your own safety rules:

-

-

-

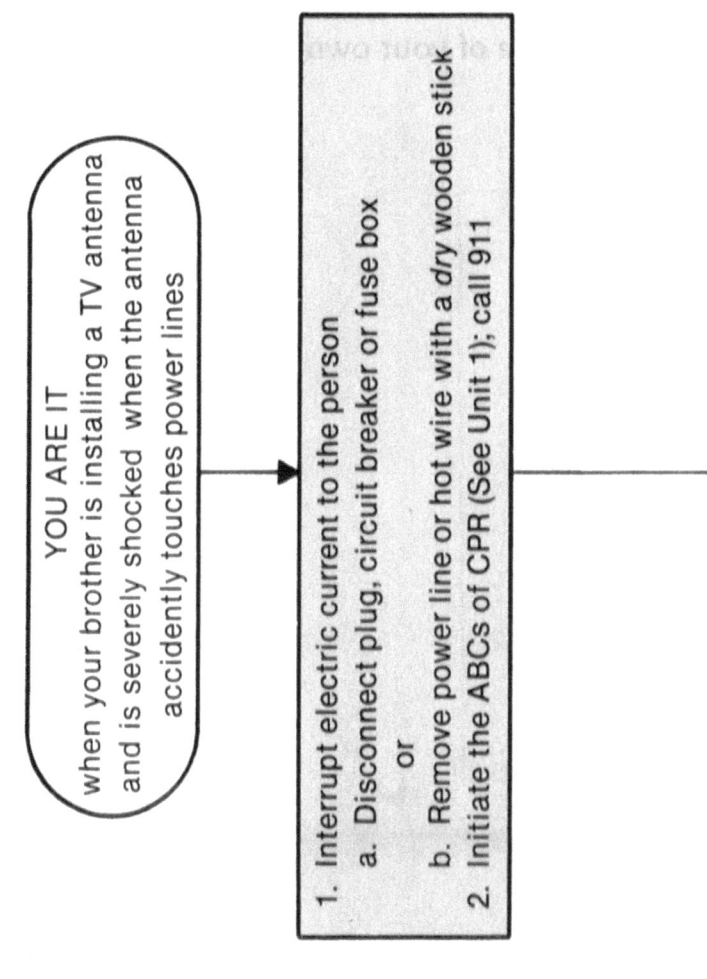

YOU ARE IT

when your brother is installing a TV antenna and is severely shocked when the antenna accidently touches power lines

1. Interrupt electric current to the person
   a. Disconnect plug, circuit breaker or fuse box
      or
   b. Remove power line or hot wire with a *dry* wooden stick
2. Initiate the ABCs of CPR (See Unit 1); call 911

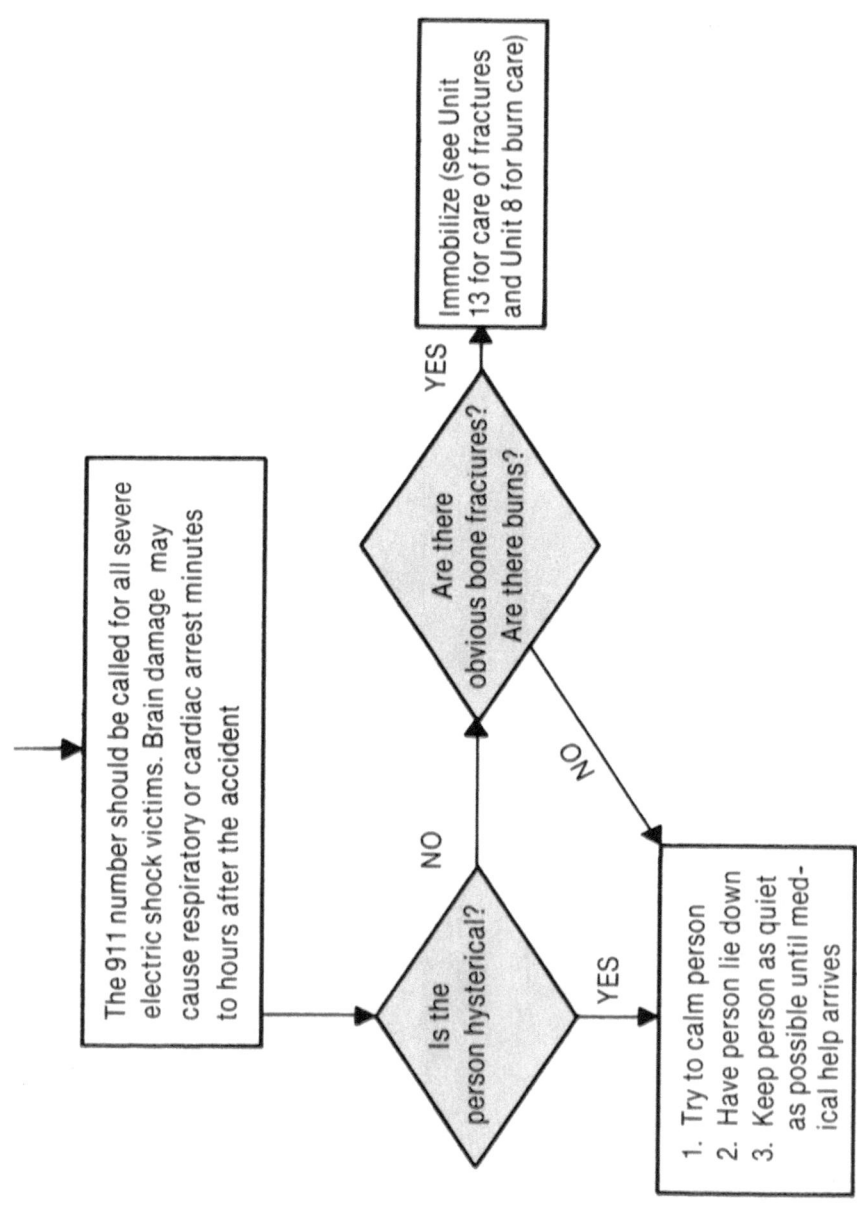

The 911 number should be called for all severe electric shock victims. Brain damage may cause respiratory or cardiac arrest minutes to hours after the accident

Is the person hysterical?

NO

YES

1. Try to calm person
2. Have person lie down
3. Keep person as quiet as possible until medical help arrives

Are there obvious bone fractures? Are there burns?

YES

NO

Immobilize (see Unit 13 for care of fractures and Unit 8 for burn care)

EMERGENCY CARE FOR EYE INJURY WHEN YOU ARE IT

Before reading this, put a blindfold on for 15 minutes. Have we gotten your attention? Good! Because knowing how to quickly respond to an eye injury could greatly reduce the possibility that a person might have to "wear a blindfold" forever.

Besides learning what to do for an eye injury, you should know signs indicating that eyes are in danger. Whenever the following signs are present, the person should seek medical care immediately without delay: (1) severe acute eye pain, (2) severe acute headache, sometimes with nausea and vomiting, and (3) loss of vision in one or both eyes.

PREVENTION TIPS:

- Wear protective goggles whenever eyes are vulnerable to injury
- Make sure machinery parts are tightened properly before starting machines
- Follow safety rules when participating in sports, such as racquetball, baseball or tennis
- After initial emergency home care, seek medical care whenever an eye injury occurs. Do not take a chance with your eyesight
- Recognize signs indicating eyes are in danger

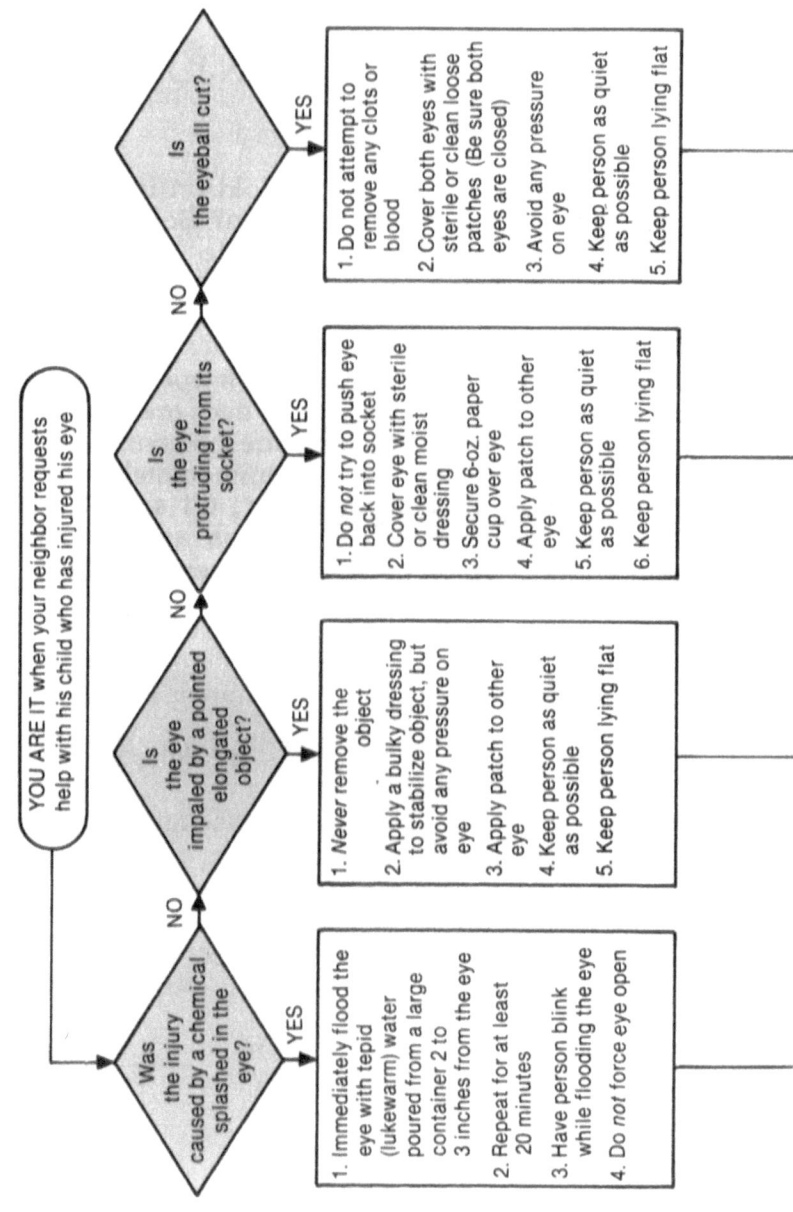

YOU ARE IT when your neighbor requests help with his child who has injured his eye

Is the eyeball cut?

NO → YES

YES:
1. Do not attempt to remove any clots or blood
2. Cover both eyes with sterile or clean loose patches (Be sure both eyes are closed)
3. Avoid any pressure on eye
4. Keep person as quiet as possible
5. Keep person lying flat

Is the eye protruding from its socket?

NO → YES

YES:
1. Do *not* try to push eye back into socket
2. Cover eye with sterile or clean moist dressing
3. Secure 6-oz. paper cup over eye
4. Apply patch to other eye
5. Keep person as quiet as possible
6. Keep person lying flat

Is the eye impaled by a pointed elongated object?

NO → YES

YES:
1. *Never* remove the object
2. Apply a bulky dressing to stabilize object, but avoid any pressure on eye
3. Apply patch to other eye
4. Keep person as quiet as possible
5. Keep person lying flat

Was the injury caused by a chemical splashed in the eye?

YES:
1. Immediately flood the eye with tepid (lukewarm) water poured from a large container 2 to 3 inches from the eye
2. Repeat for at least 20 minutes
3. Have person blink while flooding the eye
4. Do *not* force eye open

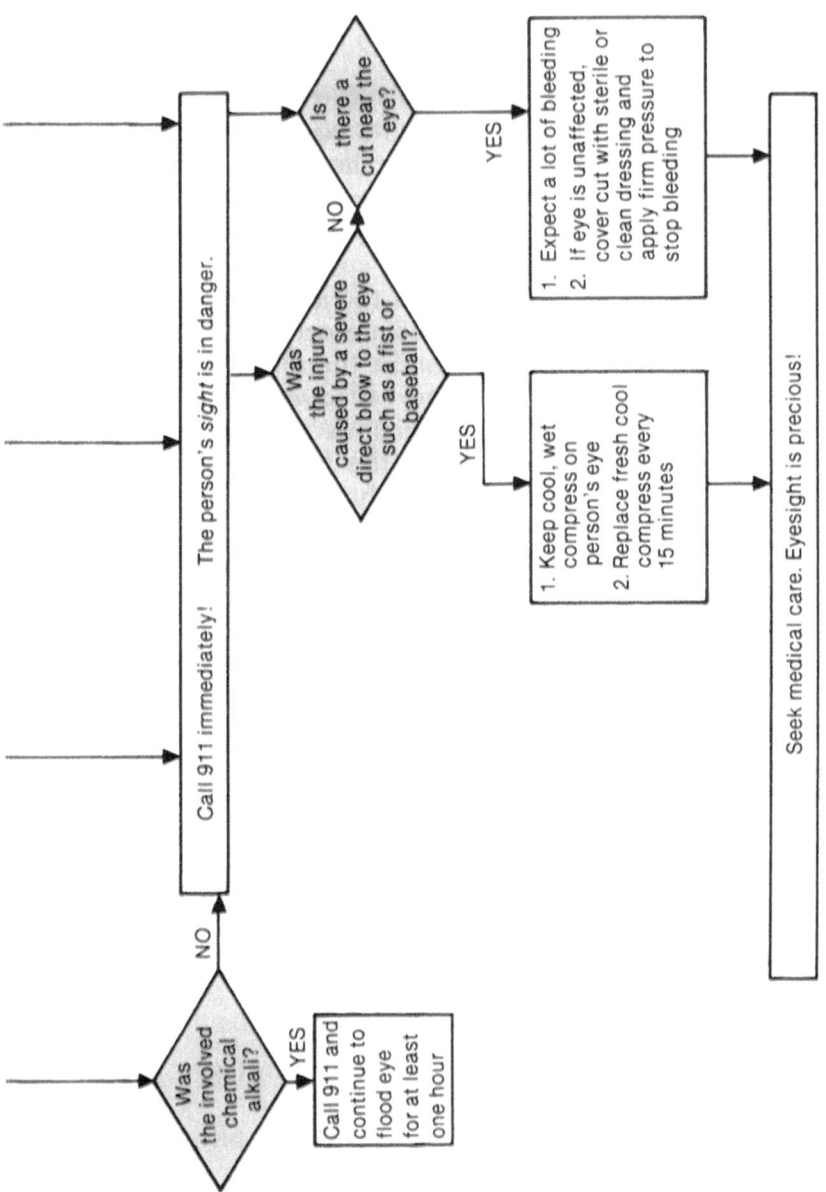

Call 911 immediately!   The person's *sight* is in danger.

Is there a cut near the eye?

NO

Was the injury caused by a severe direct blow to the eye such as a fist or baseball?

YES

1. Expect a lot of bleeding
2. If eye is unaffected, cover cut with sterile or clean dressing and apply firm pressure to stop bleeding

YES

1. Keep cool, wet compress on person's eye
2. Replace fresh cool compress every 15 minutes

NO

Was the involved chemical alkali?

YES

Call 911 and continue to flood eye for at least one hour

Seek medical care. Eyesight is precious!

25

EMERGENCY CARE FOR THERMAL BURNS WHEN YOU ARE IT

Each year millions of people suffer from serious burns. Chances are very great that you will be faced with helping a burn victim some time in your life. Of course, one way to reduce the risk in your own family is to know and practice the prevention tips.

Burns range from minor injuries to catastrophic life threatening injuries. The immediate actions taken to care for the burn victim can make the difference between life or death, and a short recovery or a long painful recovery. Immediate actions should be directed toward (a) extinguishing the fire, (b) limiting the extent of the burn, (c) establishing breathing and circulation, (d) preventing shock, and (e) preventing infection. Pain relief should be considered with minor burns.

The depth of the burn(s) (see chart on page 41) must always be considered. It is important to seek medical care for third degree burns, no matter how small they are, because the skin tissue is destroyed and will not heal. Also there is a high incidence of infection with third and large second degree burns. If there is any doubt about the severity of the burn(s), medical advice should be sought.

PREVENTION TIPS:

- Limit amount of time in direct sunlight
- Maintain hot water heater at 130°F or less
- Store gasoline out of children's reach
- Do not allow children to play with explosives, e.g., firecrackers
- Do not allow children near stove without *constant adult* supervision
- Turn pan handles toward center of stove so they are out of reach of small children

- Keep all electrical cords out of toddler's reach
- Use safety covers on electrical outlets
- Teach children the dangers of playing with flammable objects, i.e., matches
- Do not smoke in bed or when lying down on couch or recliner
- Use nonflammable clothing and bedding for children
- Do not add flammable liquids (e.g., lighter fluid, gasoline, etc.) to already ignited fires, such as barbecues
- Place hot coffee pots, etc. out of reach of children

CAUTIONS:

- Smother flames by log rolling a person whose clothes are ignited
- Do not throw dirt or sand on person
- Never apply *ice* to a burn
- Do not apply ointments, sprays, etc., to second or third degree burns
- Don't give a person with severe burns anything to drink
- Do not break blisters occurring with burns

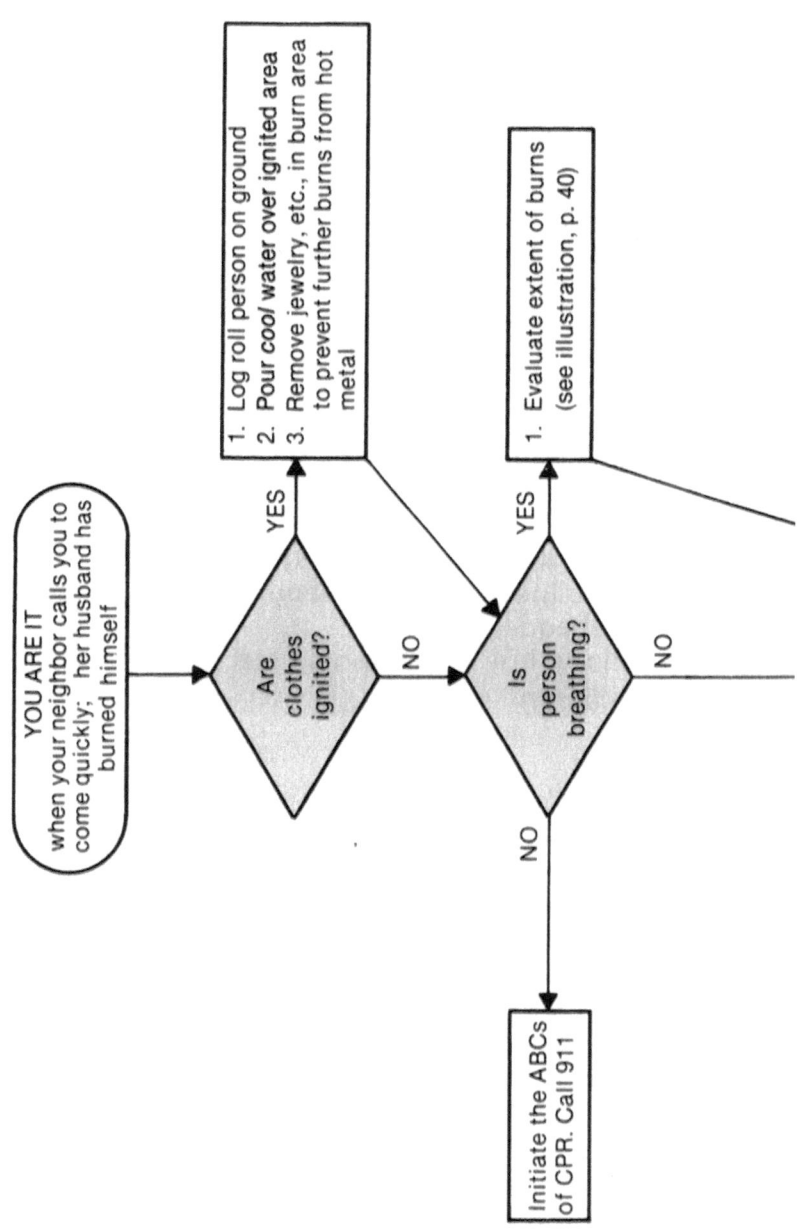

YOU ARE IT when your neighbor calls you to come quickly; her husband has burned himself

Are clothes ignited?

YES

1. Log roll person on ground
2. Pour cool water over ignited area
3. Remove jewelry, etc., in burn area to prevent further burns from hot metal

NO

Is person breathing?

YES

1. Evaluate extent of burns (see illustration, p. 40)

NO

Initiate the ABCs of CPR. Call 911

NO

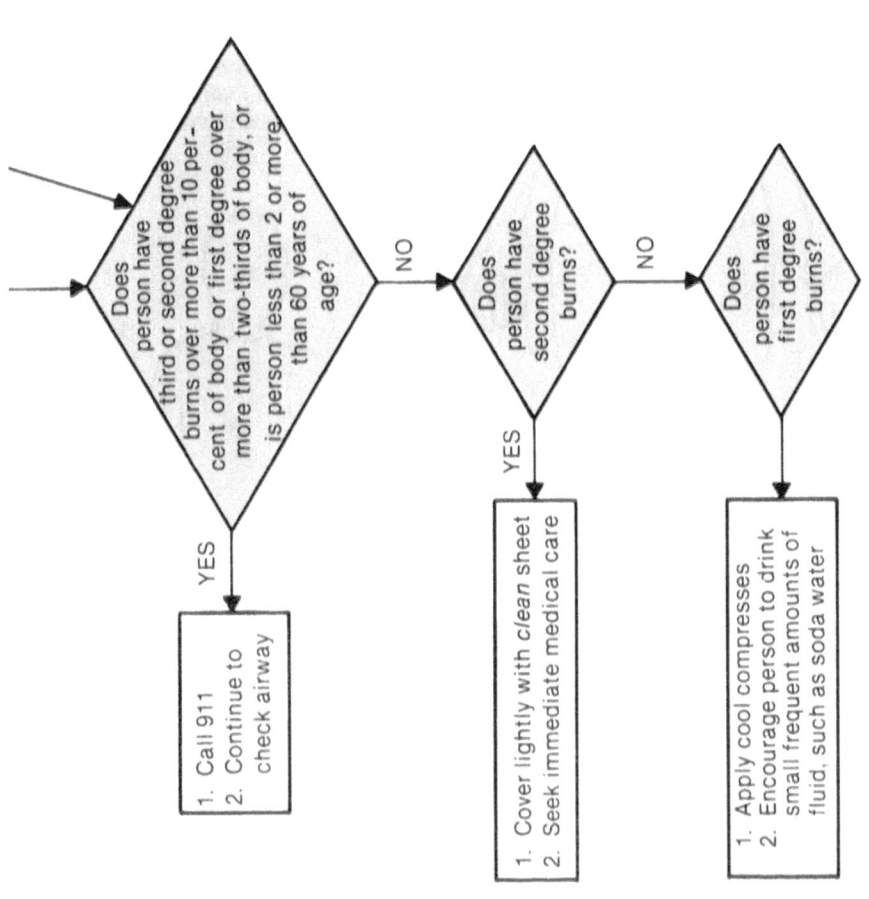

Does person have third or second degree burns over more than 10 per-cent of body or first degree over more than two-thirds of body, or is person less than 2 or more than 60 years of age?

YES

1. Call 911
2. Continue to check airway

NO

Does person have second degree burns?

YES

1. Cover lightly with *clean* sheet
2. Seek immediate medical care

NO

Does person have first degree burns?

1. Apply cool compresses
2. Encourage person to drink small frequent amounts of fluid, such as soda water

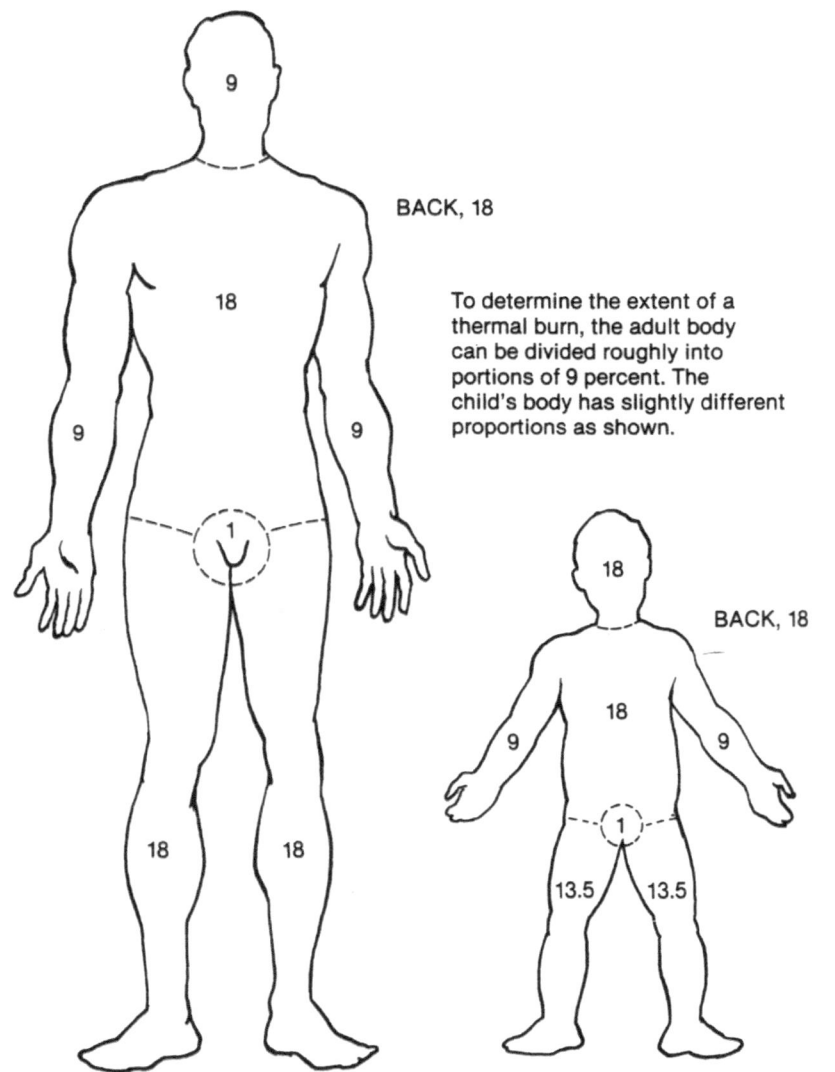

BACK, 18

To determine the extent of a thermal burn, the adult body can be divided roughly into portions of 9 percent. The child's body has slightly different proportions as shown.

BACK, 18

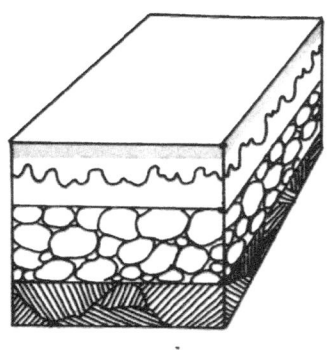

Surface Only

First degree: Area is (1) red, and (2) very sensitive to pain

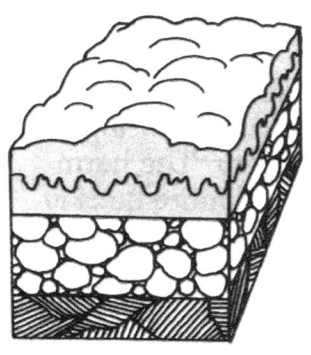

Partial Thickness

Second degree: Area is (1) red, (2) with thick walled blisters, and (3) very sensitive to pain

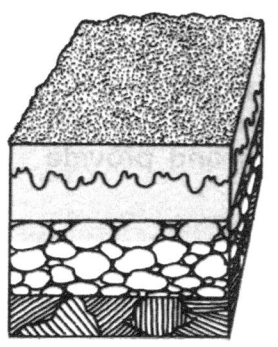

Full Thickness

Third degree: Area is (1) waxy white, red, brown, or black, (2) swollen, and (3) insensitive to pain

EMERGENCY CARE FOR POISON WHEN YOU ARE IT

A poison is any obvious toxic substance or any excessive amount of a good medicine (e.g., some vitamins, some minerals, aspirin, etc.) or *any* amount of another person's prescribed drug.

There are four ways in which poisoning can occur. A person can (1) *swallow* a poison, (b) *inhale* or *breathe* in a poison, (c) *contaminate skin* with a poison, or (d) *contaminate an eye* with a poison.

Children are especially vulnerable to poisons because they are very curious and will eat or ingest almost anything without regard to safety. The harmful effects of poisons are manifested more quickly and profoundly in children because they are small.

Poison Control Centers are available throughout the nation to permit the public *rapid access via telephone* to personnel trained to assess each case and then provide treatment, instruction and information. If the poisoning case cannot be managed at home, the Center staff will direct the person to his physician, or in some severe cases to the nearest hospital emergency room. To save valuable time, the Center staff will call the hospital emergency room and provide details of the poisoning.

PREVENTION TIPS:

- Poison proof your home by placing *all* medicines, vitamins, and toxic substances out of reach of children and away from food
- Do not put toxic liquids, i.e., gasoline, in pop bottles
- Never call medicine *"candy"*
- Never carry medications in your purse
- Do not depend on "Childproof" containers

- Warn your child not to eat *any* unknown substance without your approval

- Keep a one-ounce bottle of *Syrup of Ipecac* handy, but out of reach of children. (DO NOT USE unless instructed to do so by Poison Control Center or your physician)

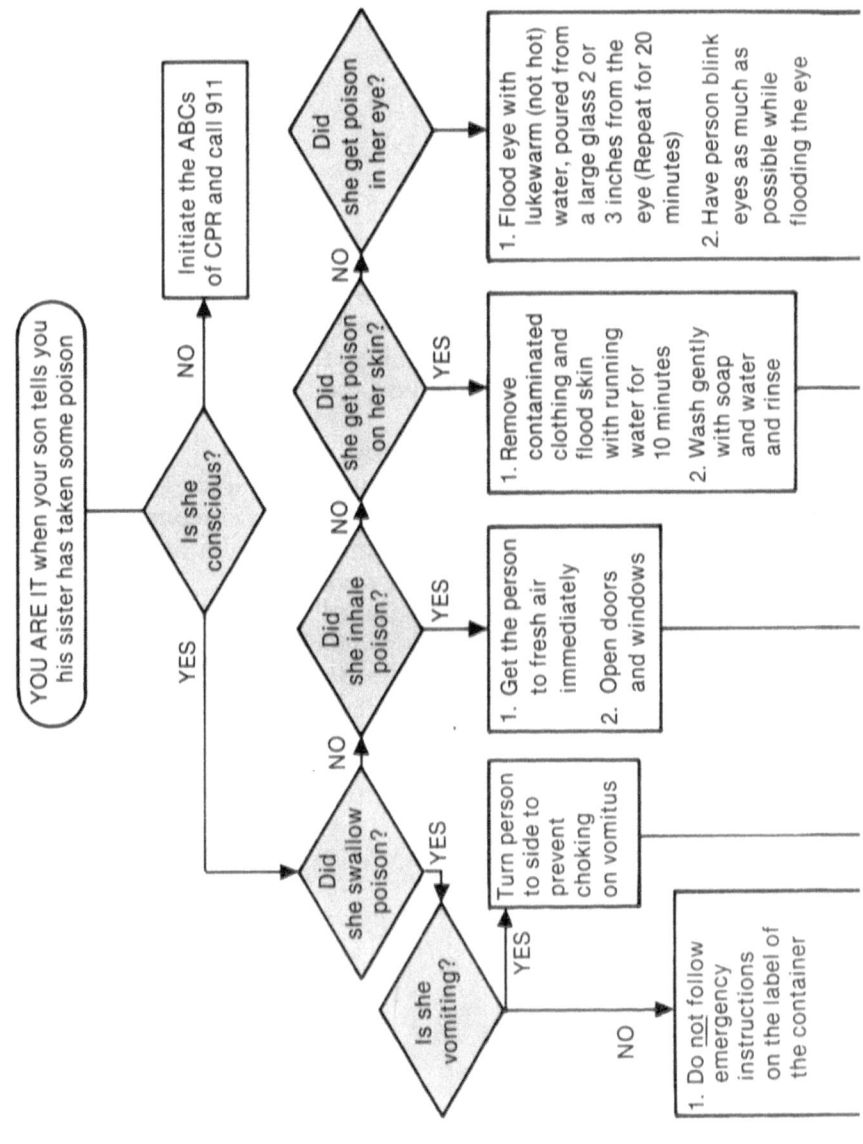

YOU ARE IT when your son tells you his sister has taken some poison

Is she conscious?
- NO → Initiate the ABCs of CPR and call 911
- YES ↓

Did she swallow poison?
- NO →
- YES ↓

Is she vomiting?
- YES → Turn person to side to prevent choking on vomitus
- NO → 1. Do not follow emergency instructions on the label of the container

Did she inhale poison?
- NO →
- YES → 1. Get the person to fresh air immediately 2. Open doors and windows

Did she get poison on her skin?
- NO →
- YES → 1. Remove contaminated clothing and flood skin with running water for 10 minutes 2. Wash gently with soap and water and rinse

Did she get poison in her eye?
- YES → 1. Flood eye with lukewarm (not hot) water, poured from a large glass 2 or 3 inches from the eye (Repeat for 20 minutes) 2. Have person blink eyes as much as possible while flooding the eye

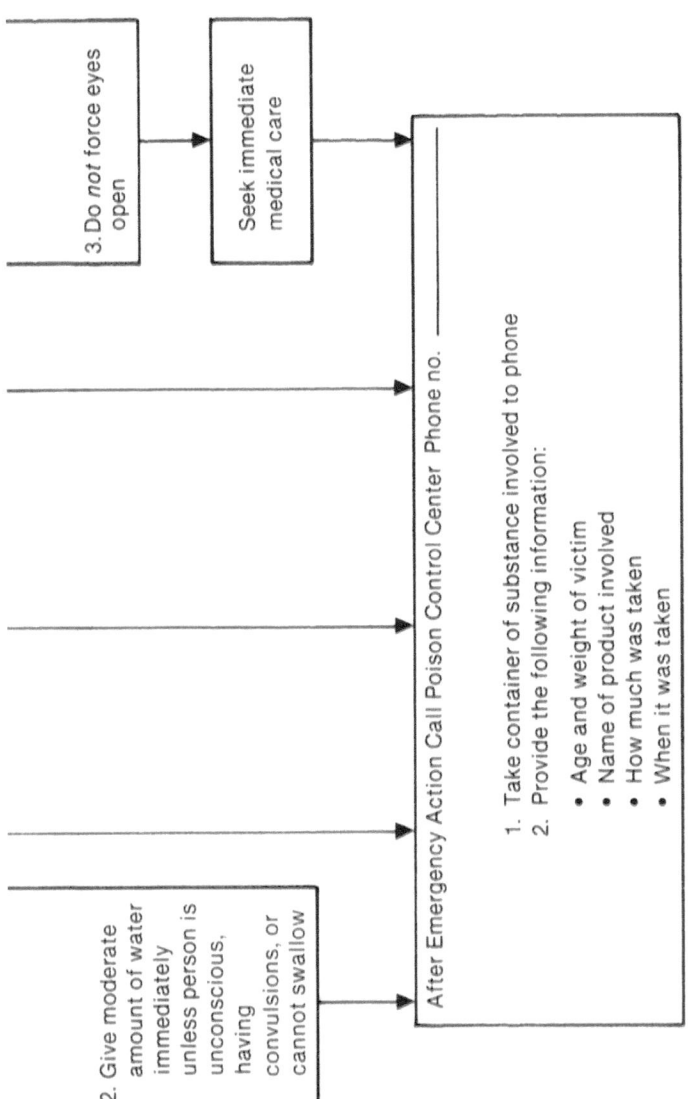

3. Do *not* force eyes open

Seek immediate medical care

2. Give moderate amount of water immediately unless person is unconscious, having convulsions, or cannot swallow

After Emergency Action Call Poison Control Center Phone no. _____

1. Take container of substance involved to phone
2. Provide the following information:
   - Age and weight of victim
   - Name of product involved
   - How much was taken
   - When it was taken

EMERGENCY CARE FOR AN OPEN SKIN WOUND WHEN YOU ARE IT

An open wound involves a break in any part of the skin. Two major problems may result from a wound. The most immediate danger may be hemorrhage, which could be life threatening if not treated right away, and infection which is not so immediate, but just as important to prevent.

There are four types of open wounds: (a) an *abrasion* is superficial rubbing or scraping off of the skin surface, (b) a *laceration* is a cut in the skin, usually inflicted with a sharp instrument, e.g., knife or broken glass, (c) an *avulsion* is a wound in which skin or a body part is partially or totally pulled off, and (d) a *puncture wound is the penetration of the skin by a pointed, elongated object such as a nail. Each type of wound has its own dangers and first aid actions; however a tetanus immunization should be considered for all of them. Medical advice should, therefore, be sought whenever a person has suffered a serious open skin wound.*

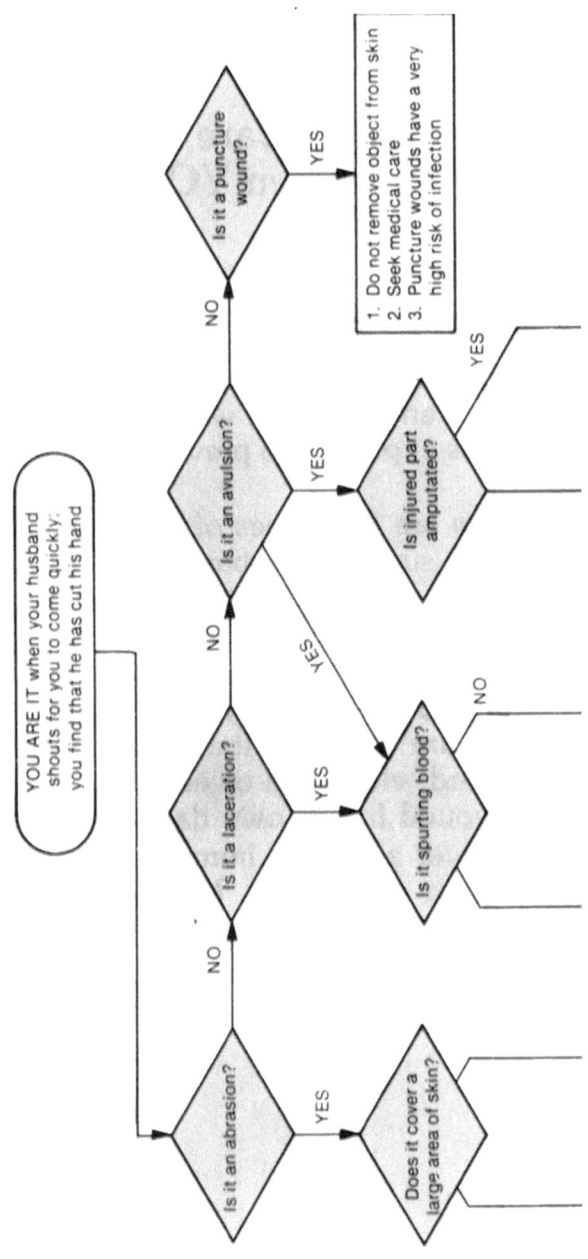

YOU ARE IT when your husband shouts for you to come quickly; you find that he has cut his hand

Is it an abrasion?
YES
Does it cover a large area of skin?

NO

Is it a laceration?
YES
Is it spurting blood?
NO

NO

Is it an avulsion?
YES
Is injured part amputated?
YES

YES

NO

Is it a puncture wound?
YES
1. Do not remove object from skin
2. Seek medical care
3. Puncture wounds have a very high risk of infection

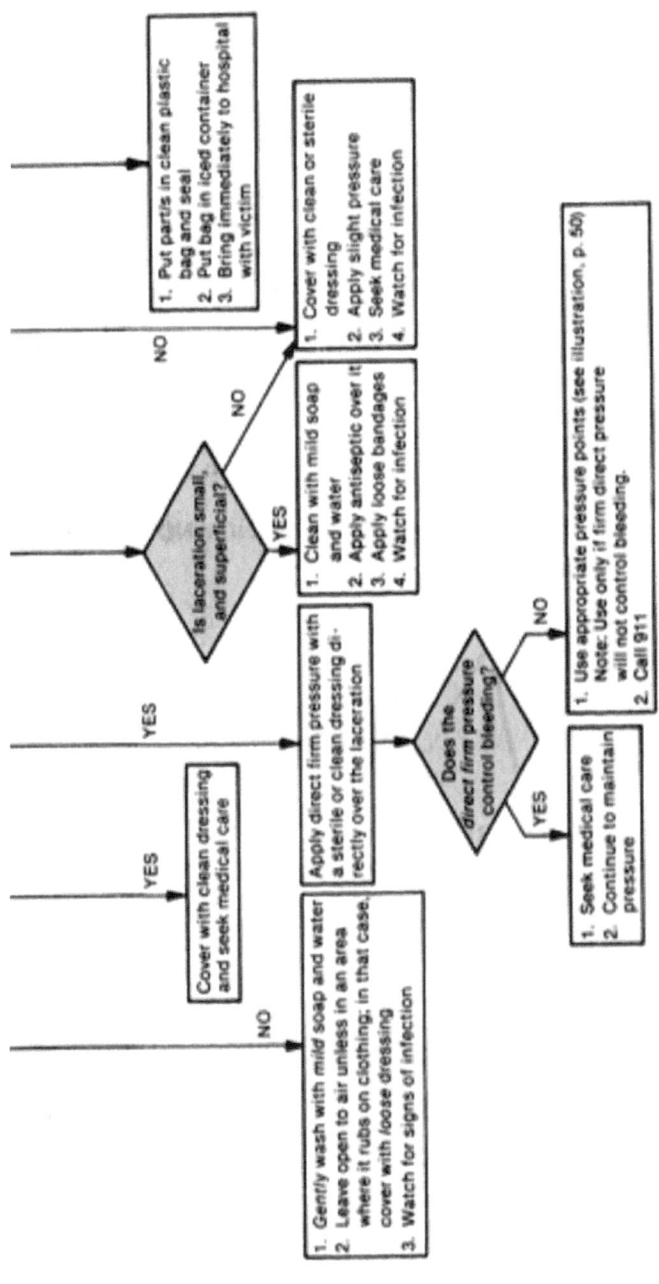

Is laceration small, and superficial?

NO:

1. Cover with clean or sterile dressing
2. Apply slight pressure
3. Seek medical care
4. Watch for infection

NO:

1. Put parts in clean plastic bag and seal
2. Put bag in iced container
3. Bring immediately to hospital with victim

YES:

1. Clean with mild soap and water
2. Apply antiseptic over it
3. Apply loose bandages
4. Watch for infection

YES:

Cover with clean dressing and seek medical care

NO:

1. Gently wash with *mild* soap and water
2. Leave open to air unless in an area where it rubs on clothing; in that case, cover with *loose* dressing
3. Watch for signs of infection

Apply direct firm pressure with a sterile or clean dressing directly over the laceration

Does the direct firm pressure control bleeding?

NO:

1. Use appropriate pressure points (see illustration, p. 50)
   Note: Use only if firm direct pressure will not control bleeding.
2. Call 911

YES:

1. Seek medical care
2. Continue to maintain pressure

38

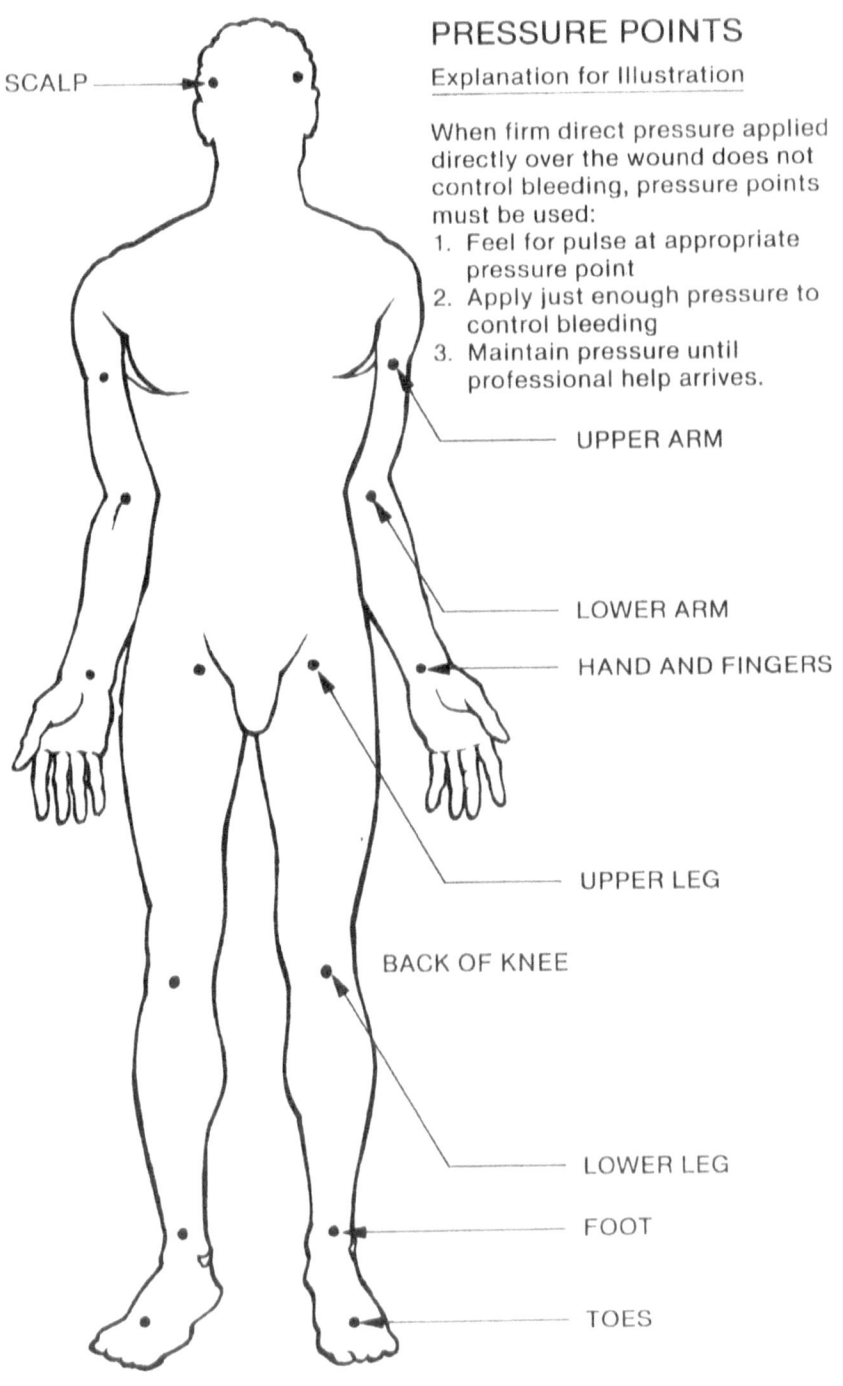

PRESSURE POINTS

Explanation for Illustration

When firm direct pressure applied directly over the wound does not control bleeding, pressure points must be used:
1. Feel for pulse at appropriate pressure point
2. Apply just enough pressure to control bleeding
3. Maintain pressure until professional help arrives.

SCALP

UPPER ARM

LOWER ARM

HAND AND FINGERS

UPPER LEG

BACK OF KNEE

LOWER LEG

FOOT

TOES

EMERGENCY CARE FOR SEIZURES OR CONVULSIONS WHEN YOU ARE IT

Seizures, sometimes called convulsions, may occur with a variety of brain disorders or injuries. They are manifested as sudden, violent involuntary movements of muscle groups. Sometimes they involve the whole body or sometimes just a portion of the body. When they occur with an acute illness or injury, they signify a medical emergency. When they are recurrent, chronic, and without a known cause, they are termed epilepsy. An epileptic seizure is usually not a medical emergency unless: (1) the person stops breathing, (2) the seizures last longer than a few minutes, or (3) one seizure quickly follows another. However, an epileptic seizure should be reported to the doctor as soon as possible.

PREVENTION TIPS:

- People with epilepsy should:
  - Continue to take their medication as ordered by the doctor
  - Balance their diets, exercise, work, recreation and stress level
  - Report any adverse changes in their condition to their doctor as soon as possible.
  - Report any seizure activity to their doctor as soon as possible
- A person having a seizure due to an acute illness or injury should get immediate medical care by calling 911

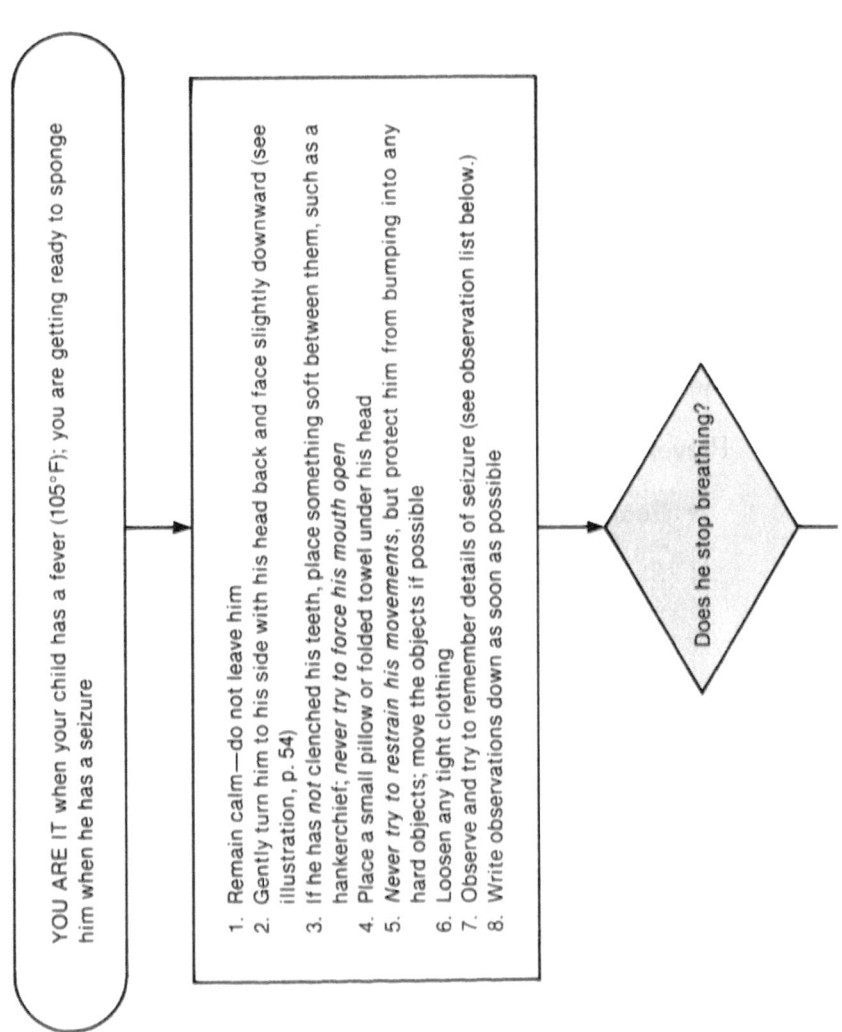

YOU ARE IT when your child has a fever (105°F); you are getting ready to sponge him when he has a seizure

1. Remain calm—do not leave him
2. Gently turn him to his side with his head back and face slightly downward (see illustration, p. 54)
3. If he has *not* clenched his teeth, place something soft between them, such as a hankerchief; *never try to force his mouth open*
4. Place a small pillow or folded towel under his head
5. *Never try to restrain his movements*, but protect him from bumping into any hard objects; move the objects if possible
6. Loosen any tight clothing
7. Observe and try to remember details of seizure (see observation list below.)
8. Write observations down as soon as possible

Does he stop breathing?

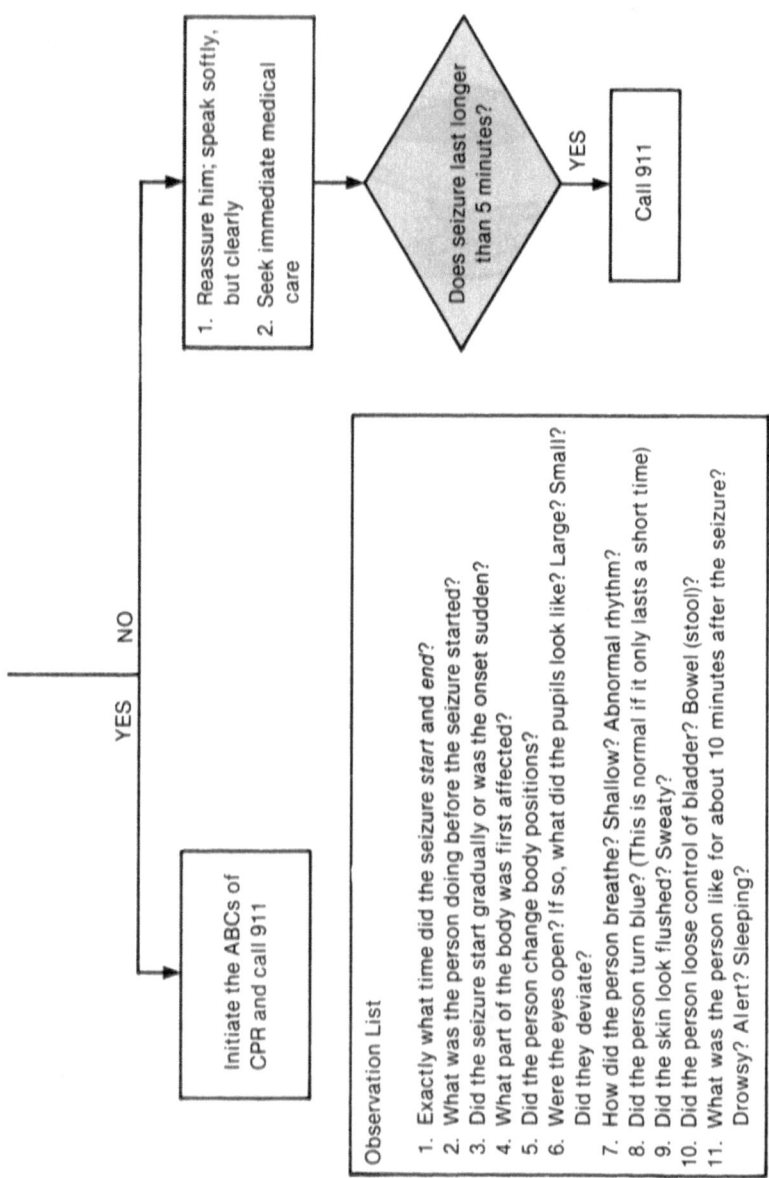

1. Reassure him; speak softly, but clearly
2. Seek immediate medical care

Does seizure last longer than 5 minutes?

YES

Call 911

YES

NO

Initiate the ABCs of CPR and call 911

Observation List

1. Exactly what time did the seizure *start and end*?
2. What was the person doing before the seizure started?
3. Did the seizure start gradually or was the onset sudden?
4. What part of the body was first affected?
5. Did the person change body positions?
6. Were the eyes open? If so, what did the pupils look like? Large? Small? Did they deviate?
7. How did the person breathe? Shallow? Abnormal rhythm?
8. Did the person turn blue? (This is normal if it only lasts a short time)
9. Did the skin look flushed? Sweaty?
10. Did the person loose control of bladder? Bowel (stool)?
11. What was the person like for about 10 minutes after the seizure? Drowsy? Alert? Sleeping?

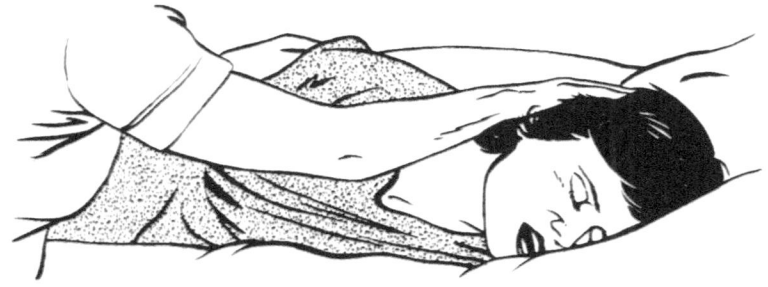

Position the person on
side, with head back
and face slightly
downward.

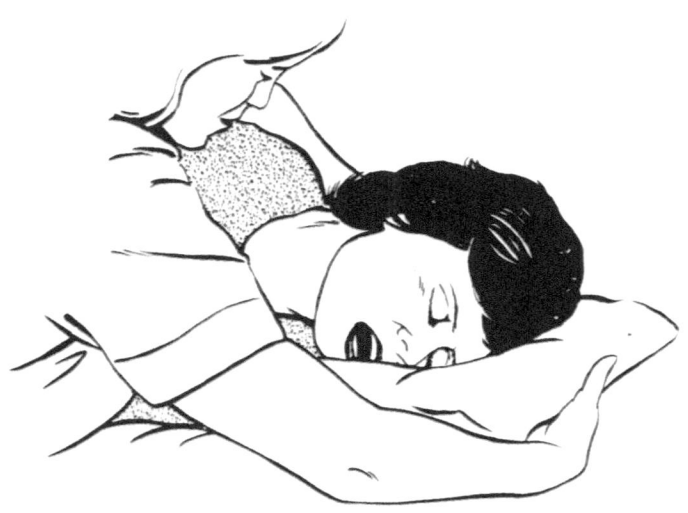

Place a small pillow or
folded towel under
person's head without
obstructing the airway.

Do not try to restrain
a person during a
seizure. Most seizures
last only 2 to 5 minutes.

EMERGENCY CARE FOR FAINTING WHEN YOU ARE IT

Fainting is a brief loss of consciousness caused by a lack of blood supply to the brain related to emotional stress, such as fear or pain. It is usually preceded by a feeling of warmth, lightheadedness, dizziness, numbness, nausea, or tingling of the hands and feet. It is usually associated with extreme paleness, cold clammy skin, and visual disturbances.

PREVENTION TIP:

- If someone complains of feeling "faint" have the person lie down or sit down immediately with head between the knees to aid the return of blood supply to the brain

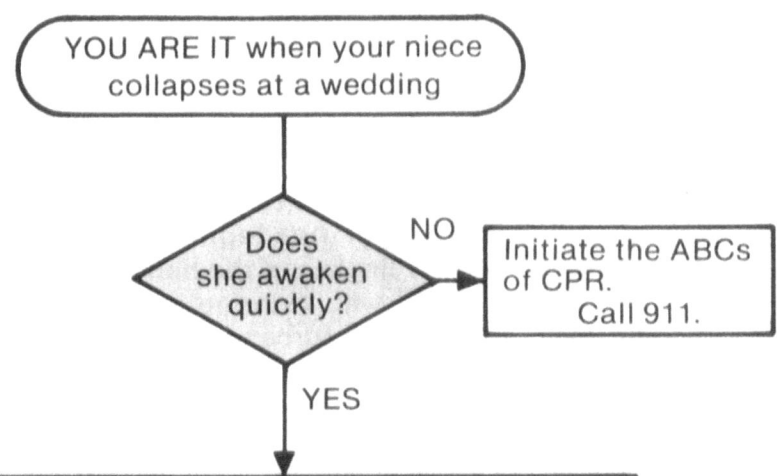

YOU ARE IT when your niece
collapses at a wedding

Does
she awaken
quickly?

NO

YES

Initiate the ABCs
of CPR.
Call 911.

1. Keep the person lying down
2. Loosen tight clothing
3. *Do not* throw water in person's face
4. Wipe face and neck with cool wet cloth
5. Check for possible injuries from falling
6. Advise minimal activity for several hours

EMERGENCY CARE FOR MUSCLE, BONE AND JOINT INJURIES WHEN YOU ARE IT

When home accidents occur, the most common injuries are those which affect the muscles, bones, joints and ligaments. Several types of injuries can occur. A break or crack in a bone is called a *fracture*. Damage resulting from excessive physical effort is referred to as a *strain*. An injury to the tendons, muscles or ligaments around a joint is a *sprain*. A dislocation is an injury which results in a *displacement* of a bone end at a joint.

Whenever an injury occurs, the victim should not attempt to put weight on the affected limb until the injury can be evaluated. A careful history and evaluation is important in differentiating the type of injury and the actions needed for first aid.

PREVENTION TIPS:

- Be aware of and correct situations that might result in falls (e.g., wet, slippery floors)
- Wear safe, supportive footwear
- Become physically fit before participating in sport activities
- Maintain a physical fitness program to promote muscle and bone strength and flexibility

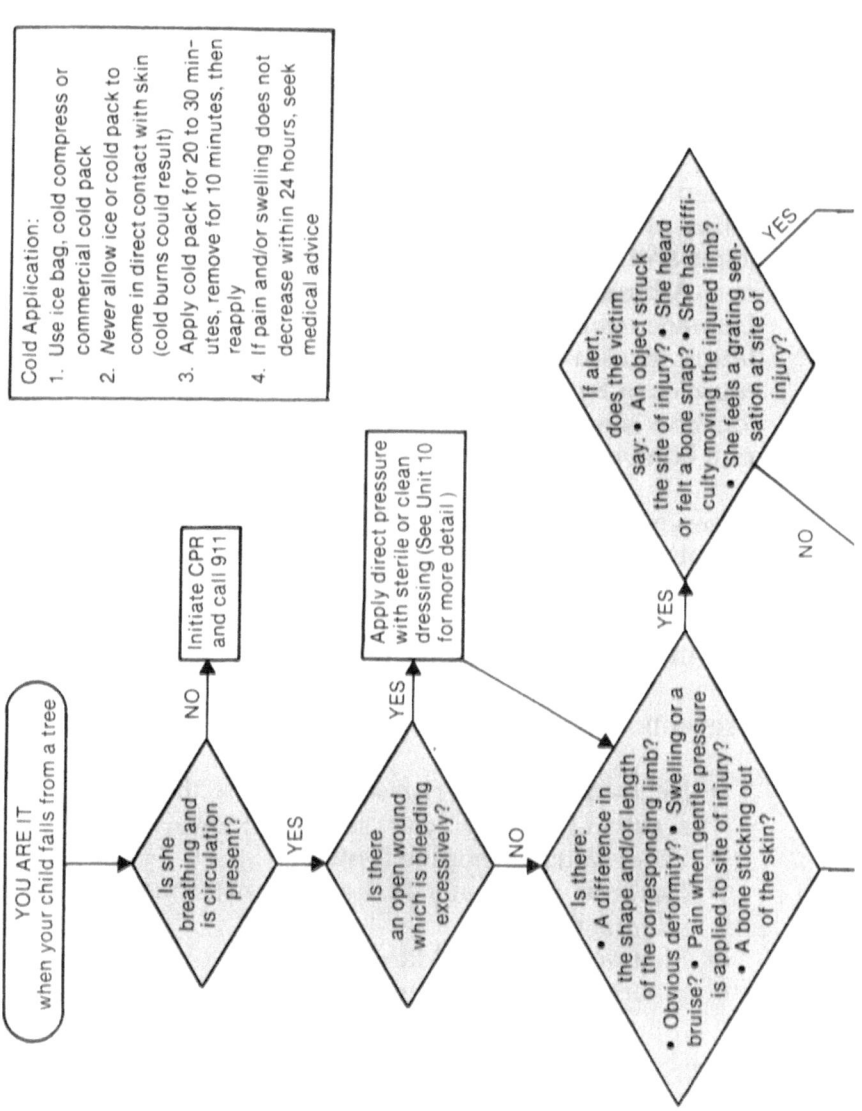

Cold Application:

1. Use ice bag, cold compress or commercial cold pack

2. *Never* allow ice or cold pack to come in direct contact with skin (cold burns could result)

3. Apply cold pack for 20 to 30 minutes, remove for 10 minutes, then reapply

4. If pain and/or swelling does not decrease within 24 hours, seek medical advice

YOU ARE IT
when your child falls from a tree

Is she breathing and is circulation present?

NO → Initiate CPR and call 911

YES

Is there an open wound which is bleeding excessively?

YES → Apply direct pressure with sterile or clean dressing (See Unit 10 for more detail)

NO

Is there:
• A difference in the shape and/or length of the corresponding limb?
• Obvious deformity? • Swelling or a bruise? • Pain when gentle pressure is applied to site of injury?
• A bone sticking out of the skin?

YES

If alert, does the victim say. • An object struck the site of injury? • She heard or felt a bone snap? • She has difficulty moving the injured limb? • She feels a grating sensation at site of injury?

YES

NO

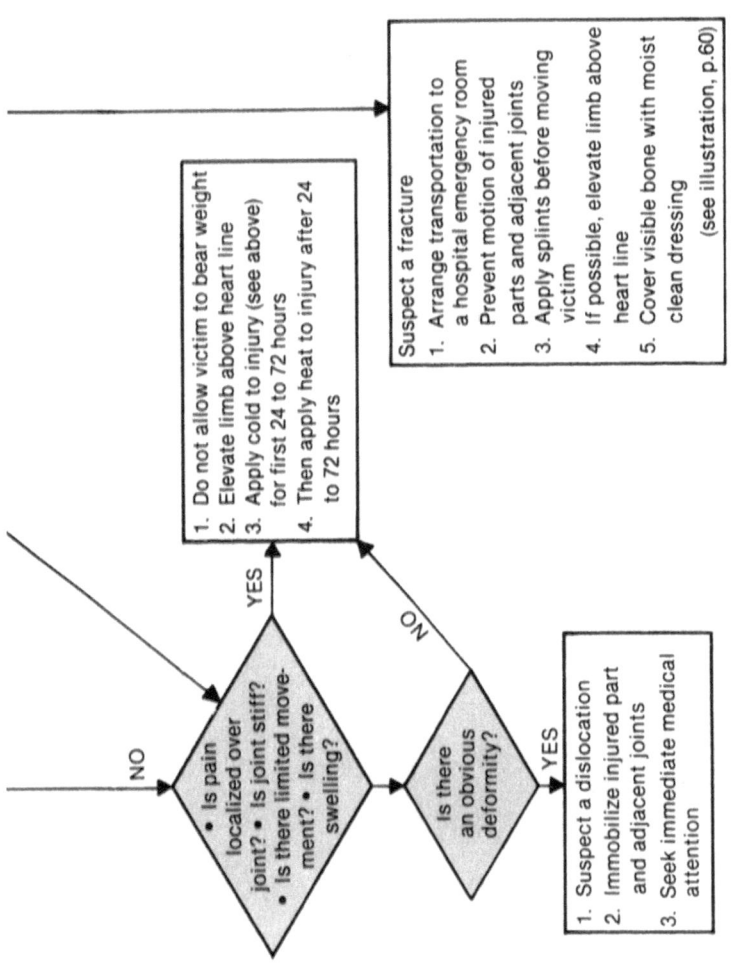

NO

YES

- Is pain localized over joint? • Is joint stiff? • Is there limited movement? • Is there swelling?

NO

1. Do not allow victim to bear weight
2. Elevate limb above heart line
3. Apply cold to injury (see above) for first 24 to 72 hours
4. Then apply heat to injury after 24 to 72 hours

Suspect a fracture

1. Arrange transportation to a hospital emergency room
2. Prevent motion of injured parts and adjacent joints
3. Apply splints before moving victim
4. If possible, elevate limb above heart line
5. Cover visible bone with moist clean dressing
   (see illustration, p.60)

Is there an obvious deformity?

YES

1. Suspect a dislocation
2. Immobilize injured part and adjacent joints
3. Seek immediate medical attention

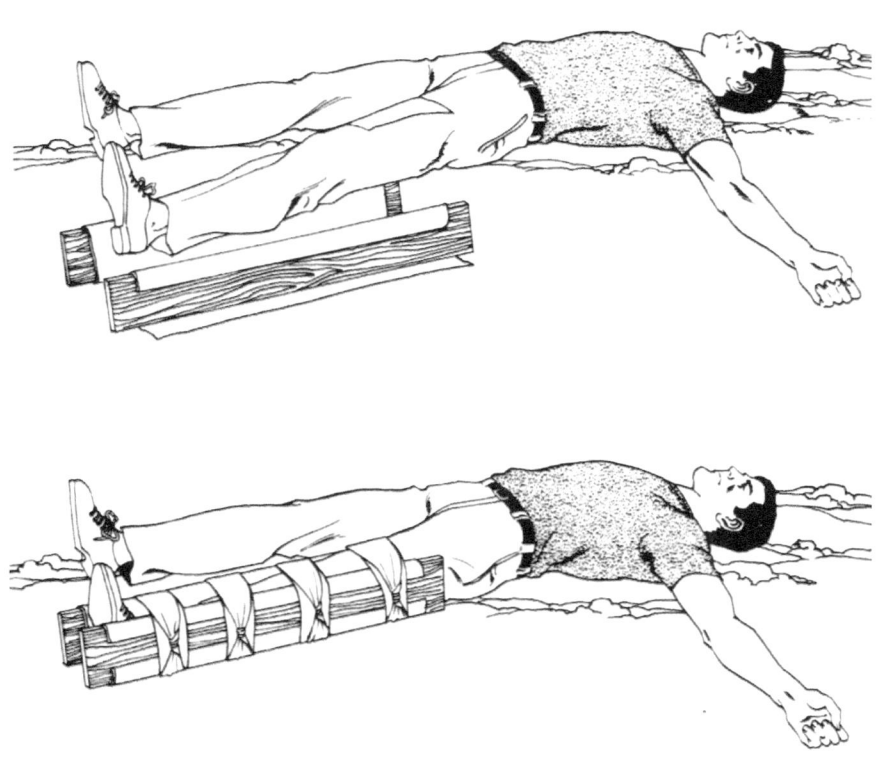

EMERGENCY CARE FOR NECK AND BACK INJURIES WHEN YOU ARE IT

Neck and/or back injuries should be suspected on any person who has suffered a diving accident, fall, head injury, car or motorcycle accident. Because the initial care might mean the difference between life and death, or full recovery and paralysis, knowing how to evaluate the injury is extremely important.

Do not move a person if a back or neck injury is suspected, unless there is grave danger such as fire, fast traffic, etc.

PREVENTION TIPS:

- Never dive into water until you have ensured that it is safe
- Wear three-point seat belts when in cars
- Be aware of and correct situations which might result in falls

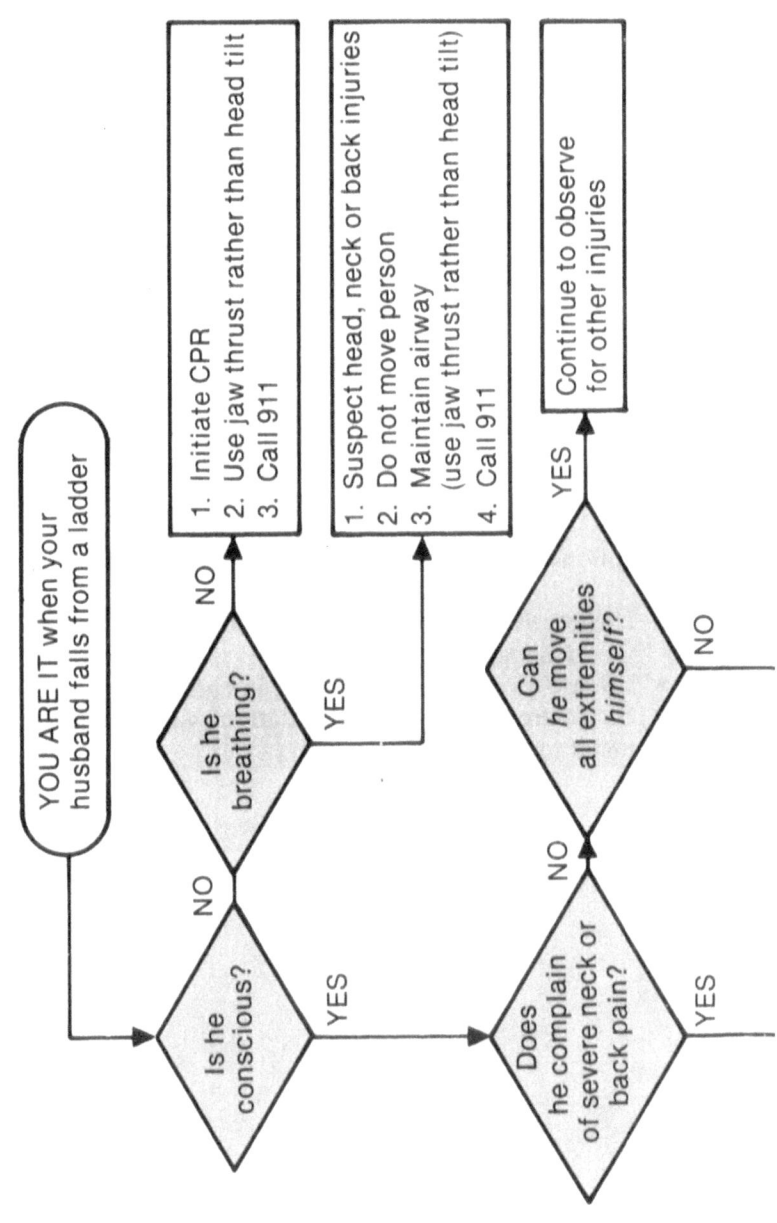

YOU ARE IT when your husband falls from a ladder

Is he conscious?

Is he breathing?

NO → 1. Initiate CPR
2. Use jaw thrust rather than head tilt
3. Call 911

YES → 1. Suspect head, neck or back injuries
2. Do not move person
3. Maintain airway (use jaw thrust rather than head tilt)
4. Call 911

Does he complain of severe neck or back pain?

Can he move all extremities *himself?*

YES → Continue to observe for other injuries

51

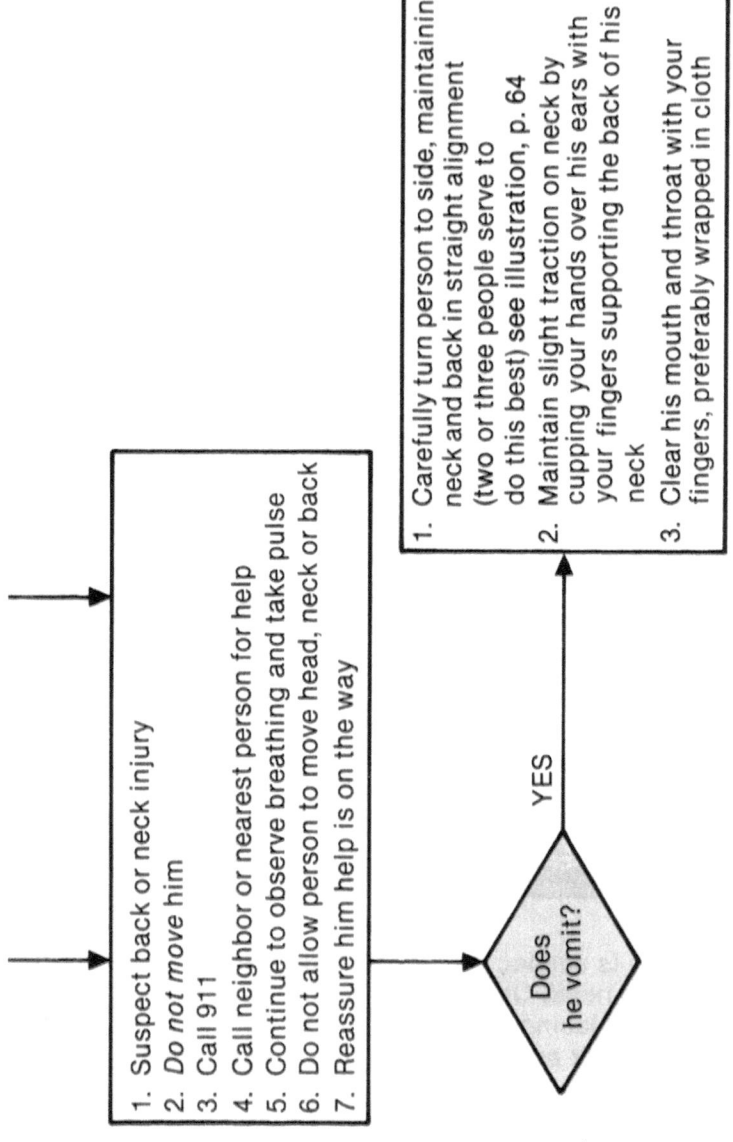

1. Suspect back or neck injury
2. *Do not move him*
3. Call 911
4. Call neighbor or nearest person for help
5. Continue to observe breathing and take pulse
6. Do not allow person to move head, neck or back
7. Reassure him help is on the way

Does he vomit?

YES

1. Carefully turn person to side, maintaining neck and back in straight alignment (two or three people serve to do this best) see illustration, p. 64
2. Maintain slight traction on neck by cupping your hands over his ears with your fingers supporting the back of his neck
3. Clear his mouth and throat with your fingers, preferably wrapped in cloth

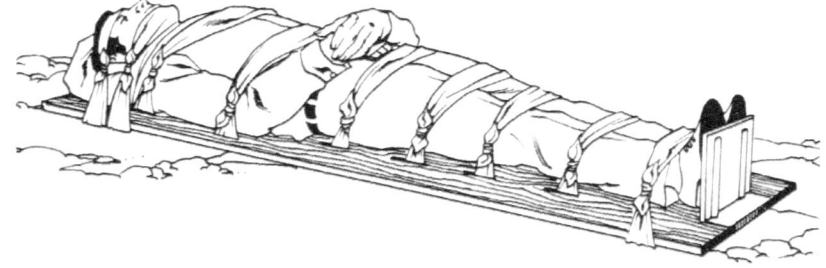

Victim should be secured to any long,
firm board with strips of material
to ensure immobilziation of the entire
body. If a person vomits, maintain
immobilization by turning the entire board.

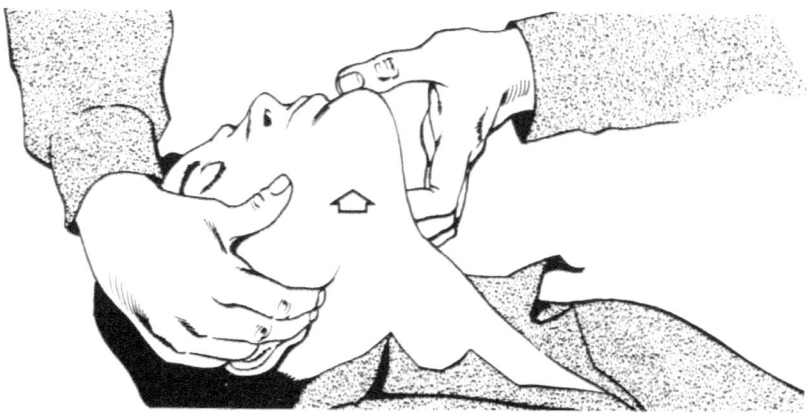

If neck injury is suspected, do not tilt the head. Open the airway by placing the tips of your index and middle fingers on the corners of the victim's jaw to lift it forward, thus moving the tongue away from the back of the throat.

EMERGENCY CARE FOR HEAD INJURY WHEN YOU ARE IT

Brain tissue is very fragile and easily damaged. Sometimes a seemingly slight blow to the head can result in a serious brain injury. In fact, any person who has received a blow to the head should be observed for the danger signals.

Once brain tissue is damaged, it does not heal or regenerate like muscle or bone tissue does. Therefore, even though thorough home emergency care has been rendered, a person may have permanent effects from a head injury. It is important to remember: "An ounce of prevention equals a whole brain." Pay careful attention to preventive measures.

PREVENTION TIPS:

- Be aware of and correct situations which might result in falls
- Wear a helmet when riding motorcycles or bicycles
- Wear seat belts in cars

Add some of your own

-
-
-

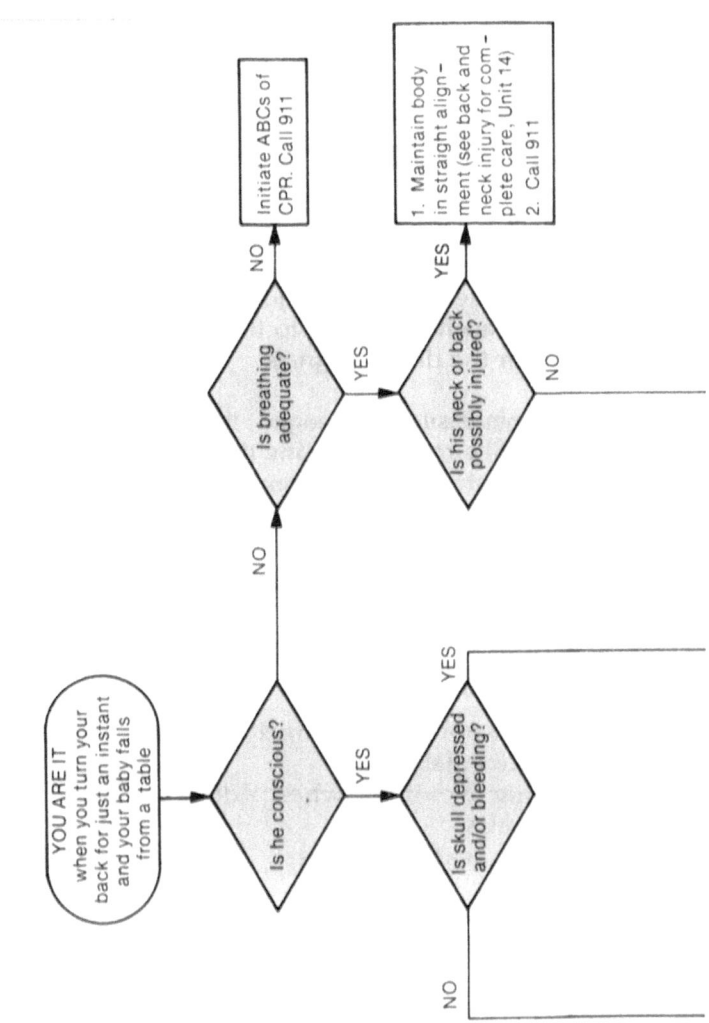

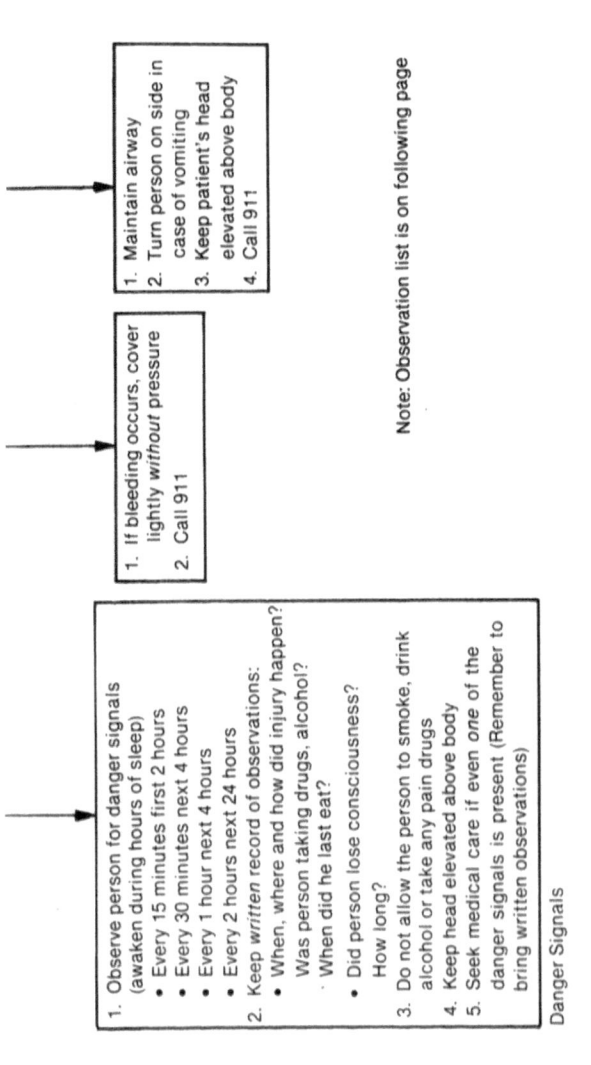

1. Maintain airway
2. Turn person on side in case of vomiting
3. Keep patient's head elevated above body
4. Call 911

1. If bleeding occurs, cover lightly *without* pressure
2. Call 911

Note: Observation list is on following page

1. Observe person for danger signals (awaken during hours of sleep)
   - Every 15 minutes first 2 hours
   - Every 30 minutes next 4 hours
   - Every 1 hour next 4 hours
   - Every 2 hours next 24 hours
2. Keep *written* record of observations:
   - When, where and how did injury happen? Was person taking drugs, alcohol? When did he last eat?
   - Did person lose consciousness? How long?
3. Do not allow the person to smoke, drink alcohol or take any pain drugs
4. Keep head elevated above body
5. Seek medical care if even *one* of the danger signals is present (Remember to bring written observations)

Danger Signals

1. Increasing drowsiness, or difficulty in waking up
2. Increasing restlessness or confusion, garbled speech
3. Pulse and/or breathing becomes slow
4. Headache continues after first few hours
5. Neck becomes stiff
6. Clear fluid or blood drips from an ear or nose
7. Arms or legs become weaker
8. Seizures (See Unit 11)
9. Blurred or double vision

56

OBSERVATION LIST FOR HEAD INJURY

DESCRIPTION OF INJURY:

↑ = **INCREASED**
√ = **SAME**
↓ = **DECREASED**
∅ = **NONE**

OBSERVATION/ TIME												COMMENTS
Drowsiness												
Confusion												
Garbled speech												
Wakes up easily												
Pulse rate												
Respiration rate												
Headache												
Drainage from ears												
Drainage from nose												
Strength in arms												
Strength in legs												
Seizures (if present, describe)												
Where began (i.e. R arm to R leg, etc.)												
Full body												
Part body (i.e. R arm only)												
How long?												
Vision: Blurred												
Vision: Double												

EMERGENCY CARE FOR FEVER
WHEN YOU ARE IT

The body maintains a stable temperature by balancing heat production and heat loss with a thermostat in the brain called the *hypothalamus*. Fever occurs when the thermostat is set higher so that the body can fight against infection or inflammation. When the thermostat is first raised, a person feels cold or has chills because the body temperature is different from what the brain says it is. Then the body starts to conserve and produce heat to increase the actual temperature to match the point set by the brain. Once the higher set point and the actual body temperature are equal, the body maintains the higher temperature by regulating heat loss and heat production. When the infection or inflammation subsides, the brain resets the thermostat back to normal. Now, because the body temperature is higher than the brain says it should be, a person feels hot and mechanisms to decrease heat production and increase heat loss, such as perspiring, are instituted. The body temperature then returns to normal.

There are some dangers to be aware of when caring for a person with a high fever. If the fever goes too high, complications such as seizures might result. Or, if the fever is controlled but the reason for the fever is not treated, the infection or inflammation might continue and even get worse. Thus, it is important to control the fever, but also to identify its cause. Also recent studies have shown a correlation between aspirin and a serious illness called *Reyes Syndrome*. Therefore, acetaminophen is recom-mended rather than aspirin to control the fever. Acetaminophen is the generic name for many over-the-counter pain medications; i.e. Tylenol, Datril, Liquiprin, and Panadol are just a few examples. Before giving any medication for an acute illness, check the label to ascertain the absence of aspirin.

A normal oral temperature in a healthy adult is between 97.7 and 99.5°F. A rectal temperature is usually 1°F higher. Children usually have slightly higher normal body temperatures and higher fevers than adults.

How to take an oral temperature for older children and adults only:

1. Grasp thermometer firmly and shake down with a snapping action from the wrist until the mercury falls to the lowest reading
2. Place the mercury bulb under the person's tongue and have the person close his mouth tightly without biting on the thermometer
3. Leave the thermometer in place for at least four minutes
4. Remove the thermometer and wipe once from the fingers downward with a rotating motion
5. Read the thermometer by holding it horizontally at eye level and rotating it slightly until the mercury line can be seen clearly
6. Cleanse thermometer with tepid water and mild soap and store for next use

How to take a rectal temperature for children and adults who cannot hold the thermometer in their mouth:

1. Shake thermometer down as in #1 above
2. Put a small amount of Vaseline on the end of the thermometer
3. If taking a rectal temperature on an adult, have him/her lie on his/her side. (If taking temperature of a child, it might be easier to have him/her lie across your lap face down)
4. Separate the buttocks so that the anal sphincter may be clearly seen

5. Insert the mercury bulb about one inch into the rectum, aiming toward the navel, <u>NEVER</u> <u>FORCE IT</u>

6. Hold the thermometer in place for at least four minutes

7. Remove and read the thermometer as above

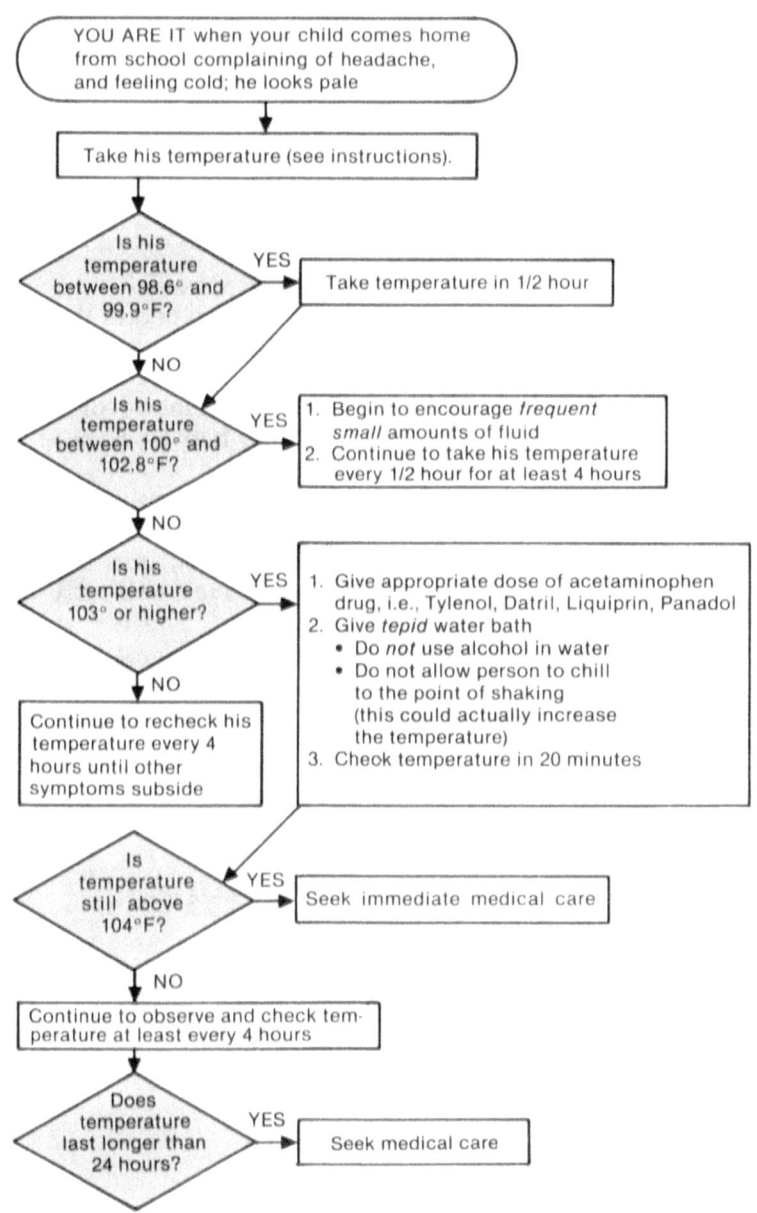

YOU ARE IT when your child comes home from school complaining of headache, and feeling cold; he looks pale

Take his temperature (see instructions).

Is his temperature between 98.6° and 99.9°F?

YES → Take temperature in 1/2 hour

NO ↓

Is his temperature between 100° and 102.8°F?

YES →
1. Begin to encourage *frequent small* amounts of fluid
2. Continue to take his temperature every 1/2 hour for at least 4 hours

NO ↓

Is his temperature 103° or higher?

YES →
1. Give appropriate dose of acetaminophen drug, i.e., Tylenol, Datril, Liquiprin, Panadol
2. Give *tepid* water bath
   • Do *not* use alcohol in water
   • Do not allow person to chill to the point of shaking (this could actually increase the temperature)
3. Check temperature in 20 minutes

NO ↓

Continue to recheck his temperature every 4 hours until other symptoms subside

Is temperature still above 104°F?

YES → Seek immediate medical care

NO ↓

Continue to observe and check temperature at least every 4 hours

Does temperature last longer than 24 hours?

YES → Seek medical care

EMERGENCY CARE FOR SNAKEBITE WHEN YOU ARE IT

There are four different species of poisonous snakes in the United States. The rattlesnake, the copperhead, the cottonmouth moccasin and the coral snake. All four of these snakes have triangular heads which is the easiest characteristic to recognize. Snakes are not aggressive and will attack only to protect themselves when cornered or provoked. If given the chance, they will quickly retreat.

Death due to snakebites in the United States is very rare. However, since the pain and suffering from a bite can be quite significant, it is worth paying attention to the prevention tips.

PREVENTION TIPS:

- Do not play with snakes
- Carry snakebite kit when in wilderness areas and more than 30 to 40 minutes away from an emergency hospital
- Know when and where snakes are likely to be:
  — Snakes are active March through October
  — Maine, Alaska and Hawaii are the only states which do not have poisonous snakes
- Be able to recognize poisonous snakes
- Before entering areas where snakes are likely to be, make plenty of noise; snakes are shy and will retreat if given a chance
- Do not apply ice to wound (local tissue damage will occur)

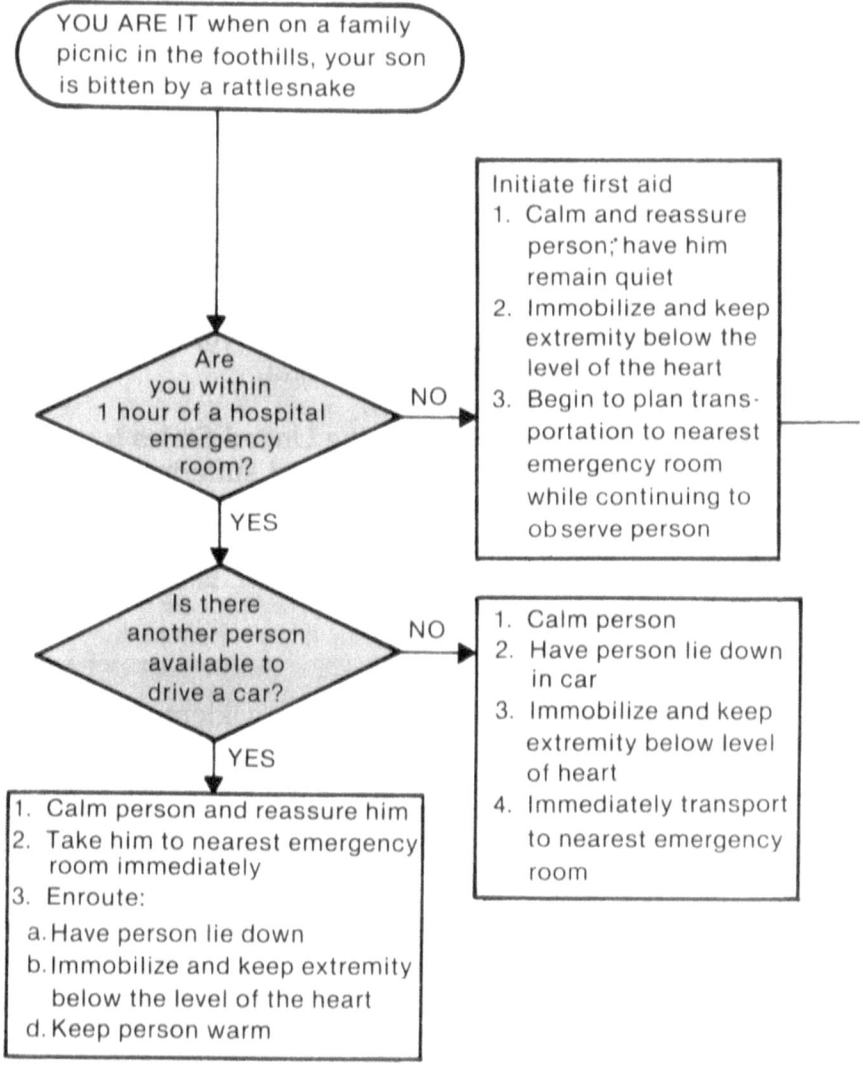

YOU ARE IT when on a family picnic in the foothills, your son is bitten by a rattlesnake

Are you within 1 hour of a hospital emergency room?

NO

Initiate first aid
1. Calm and reassure person; have him remain quiet
2. Immobilize and keep extremity below the level of the heart
3. Begin to plan transportation to nearest emergency room while continuing to observe person

YES

Is there another person available to drive a car?

NO

1. Calm person
2. Have person lie down in car
3. Immobilize and keep extremity below level of heart
4. Immediately transport to nearest emergency room

YES

1. Calm person and reassure him
2. Take him to nearest emergency room immediately
3. Enroute:
   a. Have person lie down
   b. Immobilize and keep extremity below the level of the heart
   d. Keep person warm

Is there mild to moder-ate pain, weakness, pulse above 100, difficulty breathing, nausea or vomiting,swelling at the site?

NO

Is there severe pain, swelling, slurred speech, twitching, shock, convulsions, loss of conscious-ness?

YES

YES

1. In addition to previous actions, apply a 3/4-to 1-1/2-inch band 2 to 4 inches above and below wound
2. Tighten bands so that one finger can slip under them
3. Check pulse below bands; if no pulse, loosen bands until pulse is felt

In addition to previous actions, follow instructions in kit for using suction on the wound

1. If bite is on extremity, make one incision just through the skin over the fang marks.

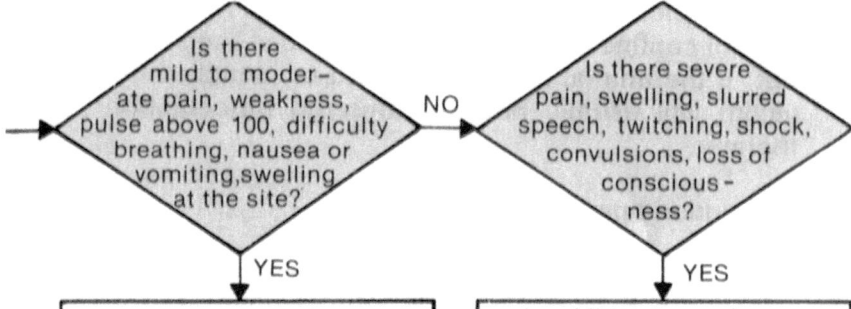

2. Create suction using suction cup or mouth for 30 minutes. Caution: Do not make cuts on head, neck, or trunk of body. Do not use suction with mouth if open sores are present.

EMERGENCY CARE FOR ANIMAL BITES WHEN YOU ARE IT

The greatest concern about animal bites is the possibility of contracting rabies, which is almost always fatal. Therefore, an attempt should be made to identify and/or confine the animal until rabies has been ruled out. If the animal cannot be found or identified, the victim will usually have to undergo inoculation therapy.

PREVENTION TIPS:

- Do not tease or play with unfamiliar animals
- If you have a pet, have it inoculated against rabies

YOU ARE IT when your
friend is bitten by a dog

1. Treat as a laceration (see Unit 10)
2. Report incident to Health Department
3. Identify animal if possible
4. Seek medical care

Beverly J. Coffman received her RN from Kaiser Foundation School of Nursing in 1959 and her BSN from San Jose State University in 1979, with a master's degree in nursing. From 1959 to 1969, Mrs. Coffman was the nursing supervisor for the emergency room, the medical unit, and the psychiatric unit at Santa Clara Valley Medical Center. She was later the nursing supervisor at Santa Teresa Community Hospital, and has been a CPR instructor both inside and outside the medical community.

Gunnar Sevelius, M.D. graduated from Karolinska Medical Institute in Stockholm, Sweden and took postgraduate training in internal medicine, diagnostic isotopes, and cardiology at the University of Oklahoma Medical School. He was Associate Professor of Medicine in the Medical Department of the university from 1961 to 1969, part of the time consulting to the newly organized Research Center of the Federal Aviation Agency in Oklahoma City. This work was concerned with stress, fatigue, and other problems experienced by pilots and air controllers, and involved using and setting standards for treadmill testing. His research involved the predictive value of different risk factors for heart attacks. He has worked as Medical Director for NASA at Ames Research Center. He was also Medical Director for Lockheed Missiles & Space Company, Inc. (LMSC) in Sunnyvale, California. In this position, he has been part of an SRI International team doing research in a work setting on blood pressure control and stress management.

Special thanks to Cheryl Cooper and Wendi Freeman, who digitized and updated this manuscript.